The Effortless Exercise System for Men

How to Get Bigger, Stronger & More Ripped Without Sweating

By Rich Bryda

Effortless Exercise System for Men

ISBN: 1492856002
ISBN-13: 978-1492856009

Published by MakeRight Publishing
(www.MakeRightPub.com)

CONTENTS

Effortless Exercise System for Men

BONUS GIFTS!

As a special thank you for buying this book, you can get the following 10 reports free at my website here:

http://WeightLossEbookStore.com/bonus:

1. *How to Lose Weight Spinning in a Circle like Kids*

2. *The 20-Second Bathroom Trick for a Super-Charged Metabolism and a Flood of Energy*

3. *One Tablespoon of this $6 Supplement Detoxes 900 Yards of Toxins from Your Body*

4. *Do-It-Yourself Face-Lift: How to Look 5 Years Younger in 2 Weeks – Got 5 Minutes a Day?*

5. *The 50-Cent Miracle Weight Loss Food You're Not Eating*

6. *#1 Cheap Supplement that Reverses Gray Hair & Infuses Health into Your Body*

7. *How to Get Rid of Allergies in 90 Seconds with Water*

8. *The Ultimate 3-Second Fountain of Youth "Neural" Fat Loss Exercise*

9. *The 15-Second "T-Tap" for Overcoming Hypothyroidism & Sluggish Energy*

10. *How to Make Healthy Ice Cream in 2 Minutes and Other Sweet Surprises!*

Effortless Exercise System for Men

DO YOU WANT SOMETHING EXTRA SPECIAL?

And here's a Super-Special Additional Surprise Gift!

Go to the *last page* in this book (after all the bonus reports) to find out how you could receive a special surprise gift.

Effortless Exercise System for Men

BEFORE WE BEGIN… I WANT TO THANK YOU WITH YOUR FIRST BONUS BOOK!

I realize I'm often accused of giving away far more value than I should, but I demand that my readers always get more than they expect.

In that light; before we get to the nitty-gritty, I wanted to give you a bonus booklet (that I co-wrote with Jennifer Jolan) right now.

For a little introduction to some of the things I love to snack on, and a sample of some goodies that make great snacks for those of us who care about our health, check out my *15 Healthy Snacks for Weight Loss: Quick and Easy Snacks that Taste Great on the Go* that begins on the next page!

Effortless Exercise System for Men

BONUS BOOK!
15 HEALTHY SNACKS FOR WEIGHT LOSS: QUICK AND EASY SNACKS THAT TASTE GREAT ON THE GO

BY JENNIFER JOLAN & RICH BRYDA

Getting Started

How often do you reach for snacks? If you are like most people, it's several times per day and may even be more if you are having a particularly active or even boring day. We snack for a variety of reasons that can be anything from feeling sad and tired, to being bored and hungry in between meals. We snack when we are hungry, and we snack when we aren't hungry one bit. Needless to say, snacking is a big part of our lives.

Walk through any grocery store and it is clear to see that we are nation of snackers. There are aisles just loaded with all kinds of snack foods. And you know you need to put some in your cart because after all, you are not going to give up snacking, even if you are on a diet and trying to lose weight. So the key here is to make sure you are putting the right kinds of snacks into your cart. That way, when you get home or need something on the run, you have healthy snacks that you can choose from.

When you think about it, choosing healthy snacks is essential to a healthy diet, and that goes for people who are trying to maintain their health and not just lose weight. Everyone needs to have healthy snack habits. After all, if you add up the number of snacks you will consume in one year, it is easy to be in the 400 to 1,000 range; depending on if you have one or two or more snacks per day. That's a lot of snacking, which means it is a lot of nutrients and calories.

Before we get into the top 15 snacks you should have in your grocery cart, let's just take a moment to discuss how important snacking is to our nutritional needs. Snacking plays an important role and does such things as:

- Fill in the gaps between missed meals or those meals where you were not all that hungry and ate lighter.

- Help keep you from over-eating when you sit down to the table and you feel ravished.

- Help to keep your energy level up so that you can get through the day.

- Help young people to sustain their growth.

- Help your body get some of the nutrients it needs, provided you choose healthy snacks.

- Give us an excuse to have those tasty things that we wouldn't necessary eat at, or with, meals!

People often reach for snacks when they feel hungry. But they also do it when they just blindly feel like doing something, often paying no attention to what they are really eating. Just think about how many times you have opened up the pantry or refrigerator and pulled out something to eat and didn't really pay much attention to what you were doing. Sometimes we even do this while we are on the phone, talking away. Get off the phone, and you may not even realize you had consumed a couple of hundreds calories!

And it's not just making bad junk food snack choices that get us; it happens with beverages as well. We are a nation that drinks a lot of its calories on a regular basis. When you consider all the sugary, high caffeine beverages that are available, it is easy to see where this would be a problem. One stop at Starbucks, for example, could set you back around 400 calories and loads of sugar. That's a snack that is calorie-packed and not offering much in the way of nutrition!

It's a cycle. When we eat junk foods or those that have little to no nutritive value, we tend to need to keep eating more and more, which gives us more calories than our bodies need. When that happens, we store those extra calories as fat. And if you are trying to lose weight and keep reaching for the wrong snacks, you are setting yourself up for failure.

Grabbing unhealthy snacks will keep your body craving unhealthy foods because of the lack of nutrients. When your body gets the nutrients it needs, you will most likely stop craving all the sugar, fat, and salt that is found in most unhealthy snack options.

There is a better way! You have to make it a priority to reach for healthy snacks, day in and day out. When you do this, you will become used to them and crave them, as well as help your body get the nutrients it needs. You will feel better, be better able to maintain and lose weight, and you will have more energy.

Choosing healthy snacks is a key to having optimal health and wellness. And believe it or not, it is easier than you may think! Read on for the top 15 snacks foods that you should have in your grocery cart and be reaching for when you want snacks.

Beef Jerky

Why eat beef jerky for a snack? One simple word: protein.

Protein is the building block of life. Eating protein for a snack can play an important role in helping you to lose weight, as well as maintain a healthy lifestyle. Protein does a lot to help keep you from feeling hungry. It gives you the energy you need to keep going, and it will not leaving you feeling ravished and ready to raid the kitchen for whatever you can get your hands on.

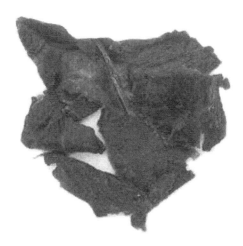

On a scientific level, proteins are important for your cell functions, so when you eat good sources of protein for your snack, it helps your body be able to keep going. It provides your body some of the nutrition that it needs, will keep you from feeling hungry, and will give you the energy you need to push on.

Beef jerky is a good source of a high protein snack, yet is not high in calorie count. You can find some good sources of beef jerky that will give you around 11 grams of protein. And the good news is that it comes with just 70 calories per serving. So this is a snack that will not hurt your waistline, but will help you with your weight and health goals.

Proteins are important to the body because they are made up of amino acids, which act like building blocks. Some of these amino acids are essential, meaning that the body cannot make them, and you need to get them through the diet. Beef jerky is a source of a complete protein that offers the body all the essential amino acids, and is low in fat. It's a top-rated snack option that will help keep you satisfied and humming along!

To find a good source of beef jerky, check the brands in your area. Compare such things as the amount of protein per serving, as well as the sodium and fat. Choose one that will deliver a lot of protein, with little fat and not too much sodium. If you can, find fresh made beef jerky in your area or try making it yourself.

String Cheese

When is the last time you had some string cheese? As a kid, and maybe even as an adult, you have likely had some. You sat there pulling it apart, string by string, having fun, and enjoying your snack. Sure, it's fun, but did you realize that it was actually a smart snack choice as well?

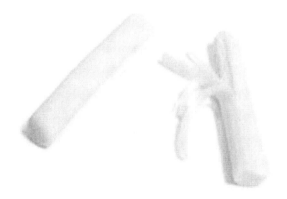

String cheese, like beef jerky, is a power house of protein. It's a snack that is going to help curb the craving to eat something and will also give you protein and some calcium to boot.

By keeping snacks like string cheese on hand, you can quickly grab a healthy snack that you can eat in minutes and meet the nutrition needs your body is craving. String cheese can be purchased at most stores, and even many convenience stores. So, like beef jerky, if you find yourself at a convenience store or gas station and need a quick snack, there is a good chance they will have some on hand. Just head over to where they keep the chilled foods and see what they have to offer.

String cheese comes in a variety of flavors and styles, including some that have more fat than others. If you are watching your weight, you will want to opt for the variety that is low fat. There is a good chance you will never know the difference in flavor because most people tend to like the low fat string cheese just as much as the full fat varieties (or at least pretty close to it).

Furthermore, string cheese can easily be taken on the go. If you are heading out to work or school, going out for the day, or taking a hike, you will find that they are convenient to take along. When you buy them, they are already pre-packaged, making it super easy to grab and go!

Apples and Bananas

You have probably heard the old saying that an apple a day helps to keep the doctor away. Well, there is some truth to that!

Apples and bananas, like most plant-based foods, are loaded with nutrients. Not only are they good for you and tasty, but they are packed with things that you can't see, such as phytonutrients and antioxidants. These things help to keep you healthy on a level you may not even be aware of. For example, antioxidants help to fight cancer and keep your cells healthy.

Apples, for example, have about 5 grams of fiber each. And it is fiber that helps to fill your stomach up and keep you from feeling hungry. There are many different types of phytonutrients in apples, which help to regulate your blood sugar. When your blood sugar stays regulated, you are less likely to feel like you are on a roller coaster ride, where you are starving one minute and then full the next, and then back to starving.

Keeping your blood sugar regulated is an important key when it comes to smart snacking. You want to pick snacks that are not going to send your blood sugar level spiking too high, or that will make it fall too low. If your blood sugar level stays at a healthy level, you will feel good. Choosing healthy snacks is a key to helping keep your blood sugar level regulated and at a healthy level.

Apples and bananas are loaded with the nutrients that your body needs. Plus, they are super convenient and easy to take on the go. When it comes to apples, you can also find a variety of different kinds, so it helps to keep things interesting. Try the variety of apples, ranging from green to red or yellow, and sample the various flavors.

A great way to eat your apple and also add some protein in is to slice it up and have it with a small serving of almond butter. The almond butter is a healthy source of protein, tastes great paired with the apple, and will help to meet those protein needs and keep you from getting hungry so quickly.

Protein Bars

Remember all that you have read so far about the importance of protein? Well there is another simple, healthy, and convenient way to get your protein in the form of a snack. It's the protein bar!

Over the last decade or so, protein bars have really taken off and become mainstream. While they were once something that could only be purchased at health food stores, today you can walk into any Target or Walmart and find an aisle filled with protein bar choices. They are individually wrapped and the perfect size, making them an ideal snack for home or on the go.

The good thing about protein bars, too, is that there are many different brands, types, and flavors. It would be difficult to become bored of protein bars because you could simply switch flavors or try a new kind. The variety is plentiful!

Protein bars will give you a hearty dose of protein and have been designed to be a perfect snack food. They are loaded with nutrition and are usually low in fat and calories. With most protein bars that are available today, you simply can't go wrong.

There are many types of protein bars that focus on different things, including performance, being a complete meal substitute, light options, muscle-building, and others. All you need to do is try a few protein bars in order to find the ones you like and that fit your health goals. Be sure to compare such things as the amount of protein, fat, and sodium so that you can choose a healthy protein bar option.

One of the great things about protein bars as a healthy snack is that they are so convenient. They are sold in most stores and convenience markets, and they can be transported anywhere. Forget buying popcorn at the movies. Simply take along a protein bar in your pocket or purse and you are set. You will make it through the movies, have a snack, and you won't ruin your diet or health goals!

Protein bars are a top pick for those looking for a quick pick-me-up that packs a power protein punch, as well as some other healthy nutrients.

Nuts

Nuts are one of the healthiest snacks you can ever have. Some people pick up the jar of nuts, look at the back label, and set it back down. They do this because of the fat content, but they shouldn't!

What most people don't understand is that the fats that are in nuts are healthy fats. So they are okay to have. They are actually good for your body! Your body needs healthy sources of fats, and nuts are one of the few foods that will deliver them. But beyond being a healthy source of fats, they are also a great source of protein, and they have other nutrients that the body needs to be healthy.

In fact, the Harvard School of Public Health found that those who try to lose weight are more successful when they stick to that of a Mediterranean Diet that includes nuts. They also found that those who eat a handful of nuts each day are better at controlling their weight.

What this means for someone who likes to snack and that needs to find healthy snacks, is that they should opt for eating a handful of nuts when they need a snack. The healthy snack will keep them feeling and looking great.

There are a lot of different types of nuts to choose from, but some are even better for you than others. So just which ones are the best?

- Walnuts – They are loaded with heart-healthy Omega-3 fatty acids.

- Almonds – They are loaded with Vitamin E, which helps your body age healthy.

Stick to these two types of nuts and you can't go wrong. Just make sure to eat them in moderation.

Protein Shake

There are times when you just want a beverage as a snack. Everyone wants to do that from time to time. But what you reach for can make a big difference when it comes to your diet.

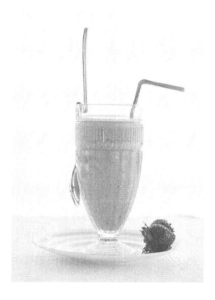

If you reach for a soda, you are usually going to get a bunch of high fructose corn syrup, which is linked to obesity. If you reach for some other drinks, you may end up with a lot of empty calories in the form of sugar. There are also options that will leave you with a lot of fat, such as ice cream or fast food shakes.

But there is a better option. A protein shake, which you can make yourself or buy pre-made. They will provide you with a lot of protein and nutrients, and they will help you avoid the high fructose corn syrup and sugary drinks, which will spike your insulin, as well as adding empty calories to your day.

Protein shakes have been beneficial in helping many people to lose weight, as well as maintain a healthy, athletic body.

To find a good protein shake that fits your weight loss and health goals, stop by a local health food store or GNC and speak with someone who works there. They can help answer questions about which ones are ideal for what you want to do (lose weight, build muscle, etc.).

Protein shakes may not be quite as easy to have on the run, unless you have made it up ahead of time or are buying them pre-made. However, if you are going to be around the house and want a good healthy pick-me-up, a protein shake will deliver the nutrition you need!

Cottage Cheese and Fruit

Looking for a healthy alternative to yogurt? Look no further than a cup of cottage cheese and cut up fruit!

Having a cup of cottage cheese with fruit is a really healthy snack. The cottage cheese provides protein, which as you have already learned, protein is important for a range of body functions and helping you to keep from feeling hungry so quickly. The fruit, combined with the cottage cheese, is an ideal choice because it provides fiber, which will help fill you up, as well as a range of micronutrients that the body needs.

If you need a healthy snack on the go, cottage cheese and fruit can fit the bill there as well. There are companies that make it in a convenient little cup, which you can just tote along with you. But you can just as easily make it yourself. Just be sure to keep low fat cottage cheese on hand, along with some fresh fruit. Within minutes, you can wash up and slice the fruit and add it to the dish of cottage cheese.

Ideal fruit chunks to include with your cottage cheese include strawberries, blueberries, or raspberries. Berries of all kind are loaded with antioxidants, which help protect your body's cells. It helps keep your body from aging as quickly, but it also helps to fight off things like cancer. Another popular and tasty option is to have peaches with cottage cheese.

Additional nutritive value of having cottage cheese and fruit for a snack include getting a good dose of calcium, as well as Vitamin C, which can help keep your immune system up.

Choosing cottage cheese and fruit for a snack is a wise choice, especially if you want something that feels a little more like a meal, but without all the calories and fat. Check out the different varieties of cottages cheese that are available and see which one you prefer. When it comes to cottage cheese, you simply can't beat this delicious and nutritious snack!

Unsweetened Almond Milk

 If you haven't yet noticed, the dairy aisle is a popular place for milk alternatives. Many people are choosing to bypass the regular milk, as they head for such alternatives as soy (bad!!) and almond milk, among others.

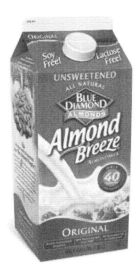

People are doing this for good reason. Almond milk provides a range of nutritive benefits, and it can be a healthy and tasty snack. In fact, almond milk has about one third the calories that regular milk has. Just reaching for it, rather than regular milk, will save you a lot of calories per glass!

Depending on the brand of almond milk you purchase, you can expect that a serving of the unsweetened beverage will only set you back about 35 to 40 calories. But in those calories comes a range of nutrition, including calcium, Vitamin E, Vitamin D, Vitamin A, and Magnesium.

Sticking with the unsweetened types will help you avoid the unnecessary sugar, as well as additional calories. Give almond milk a try by itself, and also consider using it in your protein shake, which was mentioned earlier. Any place you would normally use regular milk you may want to substitute it with unsweetened almond milk. It will save calories, while providing you plenty of nutrition.

Unsweetened almond milk is a tasty snack to have any time of the day!

Grapes

Grapes have to be one of the tastiest and healthiest foods and snacks that there is! They are super easy to buy, clean, and tote around. You can wash them ahead of time and keep them clean in the refrigerator, and you can eat them on the run with ease.

When it comes to grapes, taste aside, you are also making a wise snack choice. Grapes are considered to be a food that is low on the glycemic index, so even though it tastes sweet, you don't have to worry about them causing spikes in your blood sugar level.

Grapes also contain some important phytonutrients and powerful antioxidants. The skin of grapes contains a phytonutrient called resveratrol, which is believed to help keep your body younger, longer. It's a really powerful antioxidant that you want to make sure you get into your diet on a regular basis. Grabbing a cup of them as a snack is an ideal way to do just that.

Another thing that many people like about grapes is that they make a wonderful snack on hot days. Many people freeze the grapes and then eat them frozen on warm days. This gives you a chance to have a frozen treat or snack, but it won't fill you up with a lot of sugar or fat from grabbing a traditional frozen ice cream treat or something similar.

If possible, try to purchase organic grapes because they have been identified as one of the foods that is sprayed the most with chemicals during the growing process. Buying organic grapes will help you avoid the pesticide residue. If buying organic ones is not possible, whether because of availability or cost, then be sure to give your grapes a thorough washing prior to eating them. This will help get rid of a lot of the pesticide residue and keep it out of your body.

Grapes make a healthy snack option, providing the body with manganese, Vitamin K, Vitamin C, and fiber. Plus, they taste great and are a refreshing treat!

Plain Air Popped Corn

Sometimes when we want a snack, we long for something that we can just pop into our mouth, one at a time. This is especially true when you are watching a movie or sitting around chatting with friends. Air popped plain popcorn to the rescue!

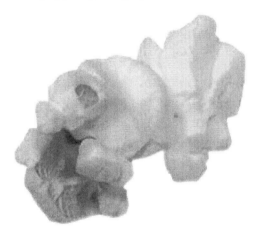

Eating air popped plain popcorn for a snack is a healthy choice that will give you the opportunity to munch on something during a movie, or just because. With air popped plain popcorn, you can eat quite a bit of it at a time, as well.

A serving of air popped plain popcorn is considered to be around three cups. The three cups of air popped plain popcorn will only be around 93 calorie and one gram of fat. But it also provides you with fiber, and believe it or not, protein.

One serving of popcorn will give you about 3.5 grams of fiber and 3 grams of protein. And since it is plain, you don't have to worry about the salt content. That's the beauty in keeping it plain – you lose all the unhealthy properties that people add to their popcorn.

Popcorn is one of nature's perfectly healthy snacks. It's what we do to it that renders it unhealthy. Adding a bunch of butter and/or salt will make it unhealthy and will hurt your diet goals. But just eating air popped plain popcorn will help you stay on track and feel satisfied at the same time.

If you find you are turning your nose up to air popped plain popcorn, just be aware that it is because you have trained your taste buds to prefer it dripping in butter and laced with lots of salt. You can also un-train your taste buds. Just eat air popped plain popcorn a few times, and before you know it, you will be craving it!

Hard Boiled Eggs

While this snack may take a little bit of prep time, it is well worth the wait. Hard boiled eggs are a nutrition powerhouse, providing loads of protein to help you get through your day!

Hard boiled eggs have only about 70 calories each and preparing them is a breeze!

To make hard boiled eggs, just put the eggs in a saucepan and cover with cold water. Bring them to a boil, then put the heat down to medium, and let them boil for another 10 minutes. Remove them from the heat and put them in a bowl of iced water. By doing this, it will ensure that the yolks stay yellow. Keep them chilled until it is completely cooled off.

To peel your hard boiled eggs, give it a crack on each side and then roll it between your hands to help the shell fall off. Then, enjoy!

Some people add a dash of salt to their hard boiled eggs, but you may want to skip that, especially if you have been advised to watch your sodium intake.

Each hard-boiled egg contains around 6 grams of protein and 4.5 grams of fat. They also contain a lot of iron, about 6 mg.

Hard boiled eggs make a snack that is packed with nutrition and will keep you feeling great!

Tuna

If you are looking for something a little different, or to help you have energy to keep physically active, consider tuna.

Many bodybuilders and personal trainers choose tuna as a healthy snack option. This is because it has a lot of protein, is low in fat, and provides some other nutritional value as well.

The key here is to buy light canned tuna, making sure that it is packed in water, rather than oil. The varieties that are packed in oil will add additional fat and calories that you don't want to take in for a snack. Stick with purchasing the ones that are water packed.

One of the bigger cans of tuna (packed in water) could account for two snacks. Just open the can, take half out, and put the rest in the refrigerator until you need another healthy protein-packed snack.

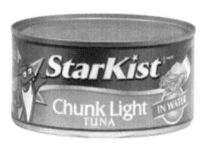

Tuna is also a good source of some minerals that your body will benefit from, including phosphorus, potassium, and selenium. There are also some B vitamins in canned tuna as well.

Another benefit of eating canned tuna for a healthy snack is that it is convenient. You can purchase small snack sizes to tote around, or larger cans for home use. The cans do not have to be cold if they have not been opened, so it makes it even that much more convenient.

Dill Pickle

Want a tasty snack that will only set you back around five calories? Think pickles!

A pickle spear, which is typically not a full pickle, is only around 5 calories. If you were to eat an entire pickle, it will still add up to less than 20 calories total!

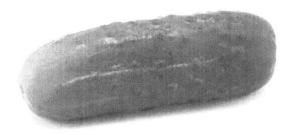

Pickles provide a tasty snack that will fill the desire for something salty, yet it will not harm the waistline because it's not loaded with calories. And in those less than 20 calories, you will still get a couple of grams of fiber, as well as a little bit of calcium, iron, and vitamin A.

A great thing to pair with your pickle if you are looking for something a little more substantial is the string cheese. The two of them together make an ideal combination. You will get the protein, along with the crunch!

Pickles come in many shapes, sizes, and varieties. When you shop for them, it is important to make sure you don't buy the ones that have a lot of added sugar or high fructose corn syrup. It is easy, and sometimes tempting, to opt for those jars of pickles, but they will have more calories and will not be the healthy snack you were first going for.

Keep your pickles in the refrigerator for the freshest taste. They also make refreshing snacks on hot days. There's nothing like biting into a nice juicy and crunchy pickle at snack time!

Black Olives

You have probably heard before that the Mediterranean Diet is one of the healthiest in the world. I have even mentioned it here earlier because it is so healthy. One of the things included in this diet is olives!

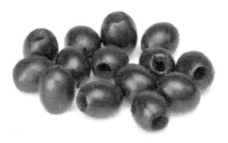

When it comes to olives, the most nutritious of the bunch is generally considered to be the black varieties. Black olives are a great source of healthy fats. They also offer the body a natural source of Vitamin E.

Black olives are considered to be healthy for a variety of reasons, including that they contain polyphenols, which are an antibacterial and antifungal. They also help support the immune system and aid the skin in maintaining smoothness.

So for a quick, yet healthy snack, reach for some black olives. A serving is usually around 10 black olives, which is only around 35 calories. They also contain iron. The one thing that you need to watch for when purchasing them is the sodium content. If you can, seek out those with sea salt, but compare the sodium content so that you do not go overboard with the salt.

Black olives are just one healthier snack option among an array of them. By keeping them on hand, you will have a quick snack option that will not be detrimental to your diet or health. This is especially true if you are craving something salty like chips.

Instead of chips when you crave that salt, grab 10 black olives. You will be doing your body a world of good!

Blueberries

Remember when we mentioned how wonderful berries in general are for your health? It's true! And it couldn't be truer when it comes to the likes of blueberries.

Blueberries have to be one of the healthiest foods on the planet. They are small, sweet, and loaded with nutrition. They have antioxidants that will help to keep your body healthy and humming along nicely.

Not only are blueberries a healthy snack, but they are also a convenient one. You can pick them yourself, depending on where you live, buy them fresh, and even buy them frozen. There is just no excuse for not having blueberries in your life.

When it comes to popularity, there is only one berry that beats out blueberries, and that is strawberries. But when it comes to nutrition, most would agree that blueberries have a big edge on strawberries. Among all fruits and vegetables, blueberries are believed to have the highest capacities of antioxidants.

Blueberries are also low on the glycemic index, so they will not spike your blood sugar levels. You can eat a cup of them, feel great, and not hurt your diet or health. In fact, you will be helping your body out. A lot!

Just like with the grapes, if you can get organic, that is the best route to take. However, finding organic blueberries is not always possible, or affordable. If that is the case, be sure to wash them thoroughly before using them to try to get some of the pesticide residue off.

Blueberries are a great source of vitamin K, manganese, vitamin C, and fiber. And one serving of blueberries, which is a cup, is only around 85 calories. That's a snack that is hard to beat in terms of health and the return on what you get out of it nutritionally!

Summary

Now you have a list of 15 healthy snacks that you can turn to in order to help your weight loss progress. Having this list will help you keep your nutrition goals on pace. If you take the time to have these snacks available to you, you will not reach for the typical snacks that will kill your diet and health. There is nothing revolutionary with these snacks. There are no secret snacks out there. Use this report as a reminder that helps to keep you on the right track.

It's important when choosing snacks to include a variety. This is why we have 15 of them listed here. You won't eat this many snacks all day, but if you can mix and match and have a variety of different types all week long, it will help keep you from getting bored. And if you recall from the beginning, boredom is a reason a lot of people grab for unhealthy snacks.

Keep it interesting and try different ones. Mix and match. Get that thought into your head and stick with it. Before you know it, with some practice, you will always be reaching for healthy snacks. They will become the norm, rather than the exception.

We wish you the best of luck in your quest for healthy snacking! Bad snacking can destroy diets. Don't let it happen to you.

Sincerely,

Rich Bryda & Jennifer Jolan

P.S. Your *Effortless Exercise System for Men* begins on the next page!

Effortless Exercise System for Men

THE EFFORTLESS EXERCISE SYSTEM FOR MEN

HOW TO GET BIGGER, STRONGER & MORE RIPPED WITHOUT SWEATING

BY RICH BRYDA

Effortless Exercise System for Men

INTRODUCTION

Thank you for getting my *Effortless Exercise System for Men*. A mere one month from now, you'll have seen and proven to yourself that getting this was a smart investment. More important, your mirror won't lie!

A month from now you'll have a totally new body.

In getting that new body, you won't sweat much, and perhaps not at all. Plus, you really don't even need to go to the gym. But still, you'll be getting more muscular and stronger. Then, each month after that as you continue to use my Effortless Exercise System, your body will keep more strong and better looking.

The Best Part

The great part of this system is the convenience. You can do most or all of the exercises at home during TV commercials. This means that you'll save money by not needing a gym membership. You'll save time by not having to go to and from a gym.

And because of the convenience of being able to work out from home, you'll also be more likely to stick with the program. In taking care of and improving our bodies, consistency ensures success. And months and years of consistency helps ensure long-term health... and a great looking body.

Speaking of TV, as you'll soon see, I actually encourage you to use this method of working out during TV commercials. So to go against the grain of most trainers and body-strengthening authors, I say "Heck, go watch TV!" I'm not going to fight you on that. All I want is your time during the commercials. That's not asking much, is it?

Correcting Common Wrongs

Throughout this book, there are some simple concepts that I want to ingrain in you. A lot of what most people know about getting stronger and gaining muscle is completely wrong.

Too many programs and concepts out there do nothing more than this: they make the simple complicated. I don't know if that's to intentionally confuse people or to sell books or unintentional.

As for me, *I promise you*, if you just go this route with me and give my Effortless Exercise System a try for one month you'll never go back to the typical weightlifting and cardio workouts. Those do nothing more than waste time and resources. Plus, they give you such little marginal gain over the Effortless Exercise System's method – and often they *reduce* your possible gains – that from this point forward your entire outlook on improving your body will dramatically change for the better.

You'll learn things that fulfill your wants and needs such as these:

> If you want a bigger, wider back that gives you the V-taper… I'll show you how to do that in a month.

> If you want a bigger chest… done, just give my system a month.

> Bigger biceps?… done in a month.

I've built flexibility into the system to allow you to choose what you want. If you want to skip working your legs, okay then do so. Not a problem. It's your body. I'm not trying to force my ideal body onto you and your goals.

Four Concepts

The Effortless Exercise System is built on a foundation of four pillars. The good news is that by learning and practicing those four core pillar concepts, you can't help but to get bigger and stronger while getting more ripped. In fact, you should write out and tape the four concepts onto your wall as a friendly reminder.

Straight to the Point!

Now, before I begin, I just want to say that I absolutely hate reading books that are full of page after page of fluff information that tells me nothing. All fluff but no stuff!

I just want to yell at the author, "Get to the point!"

So I keep that in mind while writing. I'm going to get right to the point in this book. I have no doubt that you value your time as much as I value mine. So I'm not going to waste your time by forcing you to read pages and pages of useless information just to get to the "good stuff."

I don't see the value in long books that are long just to fill pages.

As you saw from the price, I don't see the value of expensive books either. Still, personally I'd rather pay more for something that is short and amazingly informative than something that is long, boring, and full of fluff.

The value is in the quality of information. Here that information is being presented clearly in as quick a manner as possible. This program is designed for men to get bigger, stronger, harder, Alpha-male bodies.

You only need to do these exercises 20 to 30 minutes a day, six days a week, during TV commercials. You can also perform mini-workouts throughout the day for one month to transform your body and get awesome results.

If you want to put in more time than that, by all means, go for it. As with anything, the more work you put in daily (within reason), the better your results.

But as long as you follow the four core concepts, you can put in an almost limitless amount of time into exercising each day just like guys in prison. And speaking of convicts, I'm going to show you how *they* work out to get jacked up fast. They usually follow just three of my four core concepts.

And you can do that too and so much more. By following all four core concepts, you'll get better results, faster.

Okay, let's get started.

MAIN CONCEPT #1: N.I.D.M.

I learned this concept from a top fitness trainer named Pavel who used to train the Russian Spetsnaz. Those were the fighting machine men, the Russian Special Forces soldiers.

Basically, the *Neural Impulse Development Method* (NIDM) revolves around the ability to efficiently develop your neural pathway between your brain, your muscles, and your cells. By building up and strengthening the connection pathway between these three things, you become stronger, even without your muscles getting bigger.

However, because of the efficiency and strengthening of the pathway, it's much easier to develop bigger muscles as well. Neuroscientists call this the *Hebb Rule*.

The Hebb rule says the following:

> *The persistence or repetition of a reverberatory activity tends to induce lasting cellular changes that add to its stability. When an axon of cell A is near enough to excite a cell B and repeatedly or persistently takes part in firing it, some growth process or metabolic change takes place in one or both cells such that A's efficiency, as one of the cells firing B, is increased.*

Basically what it is saying is that "Cells that fire together, wire together. Simultaneous activation of cells leads to pronounced increases in synaptic strength between the cells."

In other words, if you do something (whatever it may be, say a pushup or pull-up or even non-exercise movements), the next time you do that same movement, it will be easier due to the Hebb Rule and increased neural efficiency.

This is why the core concept #3 is all about doing a lot of "fresh" repetitions (this doesn't mean a lot of repetitions per set) and core concept #4 about high frequency of movements and working out are two of the foundation concepts you must take to heart in order to get bigger and stronger.

Now, that's not to say that you can't get bigger and stronger by not following these core concepts. You can get bigger and stronger, but you just won't do it in an efficient and fast manner. On top of that, you'll probably be in a constant plateau and never improve your strength or gain muscle.

In conclusion, the Neural Impulse Development Method is just one key to making this all work. Combined with the other key concepts below; guess what? You'll be unstoppable.

Later I'll outline some sample workouts as examples of what you can do to put this all together into something easy and doable for you. The best concepts and ideas won't do you any good if you can't easily do them. Simplicity breeds activity which breeds consistency which breeds success.

Before going to the next core concept, I want you to think of your nervous system as a coach. Your system is coaching your muscles, your cells, and your nerve impulses to work together in an efficient, coordinated manner to get the most out of the team effort. How can you expect to get stronger or gain muscle when your muscles, your cells, and your nerves don't work together in coordination if they're all doing their own thing?

Using reason, it becomes clear that the more coordinated and the more efficient your body's components work together, the more you'll progress.

Effortless Exercise System for Men

MAIN CONCEPT #2: AVOID F&F

Most people think that totally trashing their muscles and going all out each set is the best way to stimulate strength and muscle growth.

That is simply *wrong*! You need to avoid both Fatigue and muscular Failure (F&F)

A complete beginner is someone in which case *any* type of exercise method used would cause him to get stronger and bigger. But if you train to failure (failure to do another rep) you will find that it is the biggest obstacle holding back progress to the majority of you and everybody else exercising.

If you constantly work out to the point of not being able to do another rep on each set of each exercise, this not only makes you feel bad and causes you to feel achy a lot, but it fries your central nervous system. When you burn out your central nervous system, you decrease its neurological efficiency.

One good way to see this is to think of a sports team. What if you trained a team to act individually? Instead of giving a strong team effort with all the players doing their job, each player does his own thing without any thought to what's best for the team.

That's an example of an inefficient team. And training to failure does the same thing to your central nervous system (CNS). It causes your CNS to become inefficient.

Your central nervous system basically kind of shuts down a bit and says "No, I'm not going to give you all I got. I can't handle it anymore. I need a break. But since you're too dumb to realize that I'm being overworked, I'm going to make you feel tired and achy in order for you to get the message."

Intensity is good and vitally important, but intensity has to be controlled and managed. Reckless intensity, such as doing all sets to failure, is out of control intensity that has a huge ripple effect on all your other aspects of training. The key to training is to master the set because doing sets wrong will have a domino effect that dictates how and when you train.

So always keep in mind, training to failure and fatigue causes your progress to grind to a halt. It's just too much. The body needs to be stimulated – not destroyed.

A Rep Example

If for example you can do an exercise for 10 reps, do anywhere from 3 to 6 reps for each set instead of the full 10 reps you could have done. I'll get into the dynamic of how this change leads to more strength and muscle in the next chapter.

The key for this chapter is to remember to manage and avoid fatigue and muscular failure. Don't seek it out as something good. Getting completely tired after each set will make your progress stall out because of the extra time you'll need to rest between workouts in order to stimulate your body and muscles again.

This results in less stimulation overall for your muscles.

Someone who manages to avoid fatigue with each set will be able to work out more often and do more sets and more total reps. The extra stimulation provides for more growth and strength gains. Failure and fatigue end up making you fall behind over the long run. You won't be able to gain strength or muscle, except in the very beginning. You don't want to be that person stuck in a plateau for years.

So pay attention to your fatigue at the end of each set and make sure to avoid it as much as possible. You do this by avoiding muscular failure.

MAIN CONCEPT #3:
L.R. +L.S. + S.R.T. = N.E.

A formula for this entire book will make lots of sense in a very short time:

Low Reps + Lots of Sets + Short Rest Times = Neurological Efficiency

This result, *Neurological Efficiency*, equates to more juice to your muscles. More muscle juice equates to you being stronger and bigger.

Here's the deal. Doing high reps is either neurologically inefficient or it burns out your Nervous System, fast. Many times both occur.

Even if you're doing an exercise that is a light weight for you, cut it off before doing a lot of reps. For example, if you can bench press say 225 pounds for 10 reps (10 reps being failure and you can't do any additional reps even if you wanted to), if you followed what I have to say, you'd *never* do more than 5 to 6 reps per set for 225 pounds.

Instead of getting the stimulation of your muscles from going to failure which burns out your Nervous System and weakens your neurological efficiency, you'd stimulate your Nervous System with more sets and short rest times from these "easy" 5 to 6 rep sets of 225 pounds on the bench press.

Now, I'm just using the bench press as an example.

I personally don't recommend bench pressing anymore because pushups and burpees are superior to it for building a stronger and bigger chest for 95% of guys. Plus, for convenience, I prefer pushups and burpees. But the bench press example works. If you like bench pressing, continue doing it. Don't let me stop you.

Inconsistency Leads to Failure

A big reason why people don't get results from working out is because they're inconsistent. A big reason for inconsistency is the hassle of going to and from the gym.

It's much easier just to work out at home.

I'll talk more about pushups and burpees in the exercise section along with the section about how convicts in prison get jacked up fast. The key thing to doing low reps not to muscular failure is you keep your Nervous System fresh and able to recover from all the stimulation.

You'll let the overall volume (lots of sets) and short rest times take care of your ability to grow and get stronger (yes, you can get stronger with short rest times).

Now, at this point I want to note. In a section later in the book, I mention how you can do one set every so often throughout the day. In this regard, you won't have short rest times. In fact, you'll have really long rest times of maybe an hour or more before doing another set.

This appears to be a contradiction, but it isn't.

What I mean by "short rest times" is if you're doing a workout that has multiple sets, you need short rest times between sets. So when I talk about short rest times, I mean within a work out.

Later in this book you'll get plenty of examples to use yourself or to work off of to develop your own workouts.

Now say you do an exercise for 10 sets of 10 reps to failure with a 2 minute rest time. That's a total of 100 reps with 20 minutes of rest. That is a tough workout and for reps 8, 9, and 10 on most of the sets, especially the later sets, those will be extremely difficult.

In fact, you probably won't be able to complete that workout with the same weight. You'll have to drop the weight just to maintain doing 10 reps for each set.

In the whole scheme of things, these types of workouts simply won't work over the long term. Your progress will stall out and plateau because this is so hard on your Nervous System and muscles. Intensity is good, but not when it's done incorrectly like in that example.

Here's a better way: With the 10 sets of 10 reps with two minutes of rest (you'll need a longer rest time with higher reps), you end up doing 100 reps with a total of 20 minutes of rest time.

Note: Most people think they need longer rest times with lower reps and heavier weights because higher reps and lighter weights are "easier." That is simply *wrong*. The weight may be easier, but it's not easier on your Nervous System. Remember, my system is all about the Nervous System.

So what you'd do instead of the 10 by 10 with a 2-minute rest time is this:

20 sets of 5 reps with 30-second rest times.

Guess what happens then?

You end up doing the same 100 reps, but you do it with just 10 minutes of rest times. And also, you do it all with the same weight since all the sets will be *easy*. You won't struggle at all. Not only that, you could do the same workout the next day because your muscles and Nervous System are fine. Your muscles are also fresh.

If you don't believe me, try it with basically any exercise. Pick an exercise and weight and do it 10 sets of 10 reps with a two-minute rest time between sets. Make sure the weight is heavy enough so that you'd fail on your 11th rep. A week later, pick the same exercise and weight and do it for 20 sets of 5 reps with a 30-second rest time between sets.

You'll feel better during the second workout compared to the first workout. The second workout will be easier to do. You'll be able to do the second workout in half the time of the first workout.

You'll be able to maintain the same weight throughout every set and every rep of the second workout. You won't be able to maintain the same weight for every set and every rep during the first workout.

The next day you'll feel fine after the second workout. Plus, you'll be able to do it all again. With the first workout, nope, you would not be able to do it again so quickly.

The bottom line is you'll be able to do more volume and more total weight in less time with the Effortless Exercise System no matter what exercises you choose to use it with. You'll be able to do all that within the workout.

But just as important, you can do these workouts more often, which leads to even more volume and more total weight lifted weekly, monthly, and yearly.

In conclusion consider the following. Let's say you and a friend had the same body and same strength. If you did the Effortless Exercise System and your friend did the traditional way of exercising using reps to failure, your progress would be light years ahead of his.

A year later he won't even be close.

You'll be way stronger and way more muscular.

MAIN CONCEPT #4: H.F.I.

Consider another vital formula from the Effortless Exercise System for Men:

Specificity + Frequent Practice = Superior Performance

Memorize that formula! You want High Frequency and Intensity (H.F.I).

If you play sports or have kids who play sports, use that formula to become or help your child become a superior athlete. Sure, there's a *little* more to it than that, but that's the basic formula and the approach works wonders.

If you want to get good at pushups, you specifically do a lot of pushups. If you want to get good at pull-ups, you specifically do a lot of pull-ups.

It's simple.

Sure, you can help increase the amount of pushups and pull-ups you do by doing other things. But that would be an inefficient way to master the two exercises.

Drawbacks

The two main drawbacks to high frequency training of an exercise and or body part using typical workout methods are muscular fatigue and burning out your central nervous system (CNS). Because of those two things, you won't be able to train often. Your body needs time to recover to perform at a high level.

That's where short rests, low reps, and lots of sets come in.

Higher reps to muscular failure absolutely destroys your CNS recovery infinitely more than low reps not to failure. However, you grow stronger and bigger by being able to handle more and more volume without burning out your CNS and destroying your muscles' ability to recover.

Low reps (without being physically tired doing them) work perfectly to imprint the movement into your CNS for strength gains not only in the movement, but also in your whole body. This results in a more efficient CNS which results in a better mind-muscle connection which then leads to strength gains. These strength gains will lead to more muscle being built.

By not going to failure, you can increase the volume of sets that you do while you're fresh. The short rest times help release growth hormone (GH) during your workout. Long rest times don't do that. You can use longer rest times than what I outline if you want, but short rest times simply work better since you aren't going to failure during any set.

It's nice to know, isn't it, that you'll still be fresh even with a 30 second or less rest between sets. But if you're not ready to do another set in 30 seconds, then you did too many reps the previous set or sets.

Not only do you save time working out with shorter rest times, you also get the added benefit of a GH release during your workout.

Please get it out of your head that you have to do as many reps as possible until you can't do any more. That will hurt your recovery which forces you to work out less which leads to doing less total volume which leads to slow or no progress.

Instead of thinking about doing as many reps per set, think in terms of doing a certain amount of total reps for the workout.

Who cares how many sets it takes to do them all?

In the other parts of this book I've given you outlines of how many reps you should do in order to get a stronger and bigger.

Once you can do all those reps as outlined, then your next progression is simply to do all those reps in a shorter time by lowering the rest time between sets or increasing the amount of sets you do. Or do both.

If you lower the rest times, it'll help more for getting ripped up and tighter.

If you increase the amount of sets, it'll help more for gaining muscle.

You can also carefully increase the amount of reps per set.

But this is the most important thing: Be careful because you can't come close to muscular failure during any set since you need to keep your muscles and CNS fresh.

For superior performance, you need to perform while you're fresh. If your muscles along with your CNS are fried, then you won't have superior performance during practice or competition. If your muscles and CNS are constantly fried throughout the week, you won't be able to practice enough to become a superior athlete or performer in the first place (unless of course you're gifted).

It's that simple.

And that is true for people trying to get bigger and stronger too. It doesn't matter if you want to be a superior athlete or not.

Frequency and Effectiveness

Now one thing I want to clear up. High frequency by itself isn't anything special. For example, you might walk a lot, but somehow this frequency of walking doesn't make your legs big and strong.

Why is that?

It's because walking isn't very intense. Frequency needs to be teamed up with intensity. Once an exercise becomes too easy for you, you need to graduate to another exercise or figure out a way to make that exercise more intense.

Think of the following:

- Are people who walk a lot big and strong, generally speaking? No.

- Are people who jog a lot big and strong, generally speaking? No.

- Are people who sprint often big and strong, generally speaking? Yes!

The Difference

Sprinting is intense but walking and jogging are not intense. So it doesn't matter how often you do something that isn't intense enough to elicit adaptation from your body.

Now, maybe your goal isn't to become as big and strong as possible. Maybe you just want to stay in shape. Fine, just simply lower the intensity level of what you're doing. You're still building neurological efficiency into your body and muscles, but you're not building it in a way to elicit more strength and bigger muscles.

Just keep this in mind: Training to muscular failure with high reps results in no long-term *progress*.

Muscle Recovery

There's one other related issue we need to discuss.

It's a myth that it takes your muscles two to four days to recover and get stronger. The reason why most people think that is because they train wrongly. They're training to failure too often (maybe every set). They do as many repetitions as possible until they can't do any more for the set.

Beating the hell out of your body may lead to gains and adaptations early on, but over the long-term your body will tap out and not go along for that ride. And this is why they can't progress.

They can't get in the volume of work they need to stimulate strength and growth because the way they're training forces them to train each muscle group only once or twice a week. Bulgarian Olympic lifters are some of the strongest people in the world. They train up to 28 times a week. Yes, 28 times!

How can they do this and still be some of the strongest people in the world? Simple (and now obvious): They don't train to failure.

They lift heavy, but they don't lift their maximum weight. They also don't lift until they can't lift the weight again. They cut their sets short and do short workouts to keep their bodies fresh and their recovery minimal. Understand this.

Never destroy yourself doing a set. Don't go all out on a set. You need intensity, so you need the set to be kind of hard, but don't push yourself too much. Instead let the set be part of a bigger picture. Let the accumulated volume of your sets take care of your strength increases and growth.

By the way, if you just wanted to gain strength and minimize the chance of gaining muscle, what you'd do is just increase your rest time. The reason for this is because longer rest times do two things: longer rest times lower and also limit the release of growth hormone (GH) during your workouts. Since growth hormone is a key hormone for gaining muscle, you're then reducing your ability to gain muscle.

Also, longer rest times mean less total workout volume overall in a given timeframe. Since there is less stimulation of your muscles, they have less reason to grow. So always keep that in mind.

You can use the Effortless Exercise System to gain both strength and muscle or you can strictly use it to gain just strength. It's up to you how you use these concepts and this method.

Anyway, the final thought for this chapter is to remember that everything about the Effortless Exercise Method revolves around each set being easy. Easy, but with intensity. The easiness comes from you stopping the set short before it becomes hard.

The accumulated amount of work you do from all these easy sets combined with your ability to do them more often will easily surpass any results you get from doing fewer, harder sets that wipe you out.

Fortunately, a simple test tells you if you were successful or not: If your mind doesn't feel energized after you finish a workout, then you did something wrong.

THE EXERCISES

You can use the Effortless Exercise System with any exercise.

So you *don't* need to use the exercises listed below if you don't want to. You also don't need to focus on doing these exercise and instead can use them as supplemental workouts that you do at home. The main reason I'm focusing on the exercise below is because you can do them at home and they're proven to work good with this system.

As long as you're not hung up on having a huge bench press, squat, or whatever else, these exercises below are basically all you need to have a great body. With these exercises you'll also build functional strength that allows you to control your body.

A lot of times, guys that are weight room strong are functionally weak. If you can't move your body through space like in a pull-up or pushup, your strength is mostly useless doing everyday normal things. Besides, these bodyweight exercises actually do contribute to getting stronger at lifts involving weights.

Give these a try using the parameters of the system and you won't be disappointed.

Pushups

There is simply nothing better than the pushup for building an impressive chest. And yes, pushups are better than bench pressing!

The problem is that most guys don't do pushups correctly.

That's the main reason why people don't think pushups are any good for the chest.

Here's how to do pushups correctly:

- Position your hands wider than shoulder width apart.

This puts greater emphasis on your chest rather than your triceps.

- Brace your abs tightly.

Your abs can't touch the ground before your chest does. In fact, the chest is the only part of your upper body that should actually touch the ground.

- Always try to pull your hands together as you're pushing up.

What this does is it creates massive chest activation. You won't actually pull your hands together. You just need to mentally try to because it forces you to flex your chest as you're pushing yourself up.

- Push yourself up as high as possible.

No explanation is needed for this. The higher you go while mentally trying to pull your hands together, the more activation you get in your chest.

- Once you're able to do 20 of these types of pushup (these are harder than the normal way people do pushups), then start elevating your feet up on something like a chair, a couch, or a bed.

This will make it harder and is a natural progression.

- Once you're able to do 20 feet-elevated pushups, do clap pushups with your feet elevated. Just clap your hands. It sounds easy, but it's not.

Those six steps are how you do pushups properly.

Now let me explain a little more. First, you're going to test yourself doing these pushups to see how many you can do until failure. Once you find out how many that is, then you'll do sets of 1/3 to 1/2 of your maximum number of pushups.

For example, say you can do 20 total pushups and no more on a single maximum set to failure. Then you'll end up doing sets of 6 to 10 pushups for the day. I'll get into this more in the sample workout programs and mini-workouts.

If you can only do 10 total pushups like this until failure, then you do sets of 3 to 5 pushups. This way, you stay fresh and keep your rest times short (if you're doing mini-workouts). If you're not doing mini-workouts and just doing sets periodically throughout the day (say once every hour or so), then you can stick with half your maximum reps per set.

So, if you did that and your maximum amount of pushups is 10, you'd do five per set. We'll get into this further shortly.

For now I'll just leave you with something you need to keep in mind. You'll need to do 100 of these pushups a day, every day, for a month. It doesn't matter how many sets you do them in, just focus on doing 100 total reps and not going to failure. Once you do that for a month, reevaluate yourself by doing a set of pushups to failure to see your progress and see if you graduate to the next level of pushups.

But the idea is to easily do 100 pushups a day, 6 to 7 days a week, every week.

I'll show you how to easily fit that into a busy schedule.

You'll be amazed at how much your chest *"blows up"* from doing 100 simple pushups every day for a month!

Pull-Ups

Pull-ups are an awesome exercise. If you want a big, wide back, pull-ups are your ticket.

Unfortunately, a lot of people don't have a pull-up station at home to do them. If you don't have that equipment, I'm encouraging you to get it. Do a search on the internet or go to your local sporting goods store. They should cost $100 to $200 and for anyone who wants to improve his body they're well worth it.

Note: If you go to a gym, maybe stop going and spend the money you save on a pull-up station. It'll be one of the best investments you ever make in yourself.

I'm assuming you know what pull-ups are, but just in case you don't: Pull-ups are simply hanging from a bar (with your palms facing away from you) and pulling yourself up so your chin goes above the bar.

The two keys to pull-ups follow.

- Focus on pulling with your pinky.

What I mean by that... pull yourself up and put more focus on the pulling with the outer part of your hand (by the pinky).

This activates way more lat muscles (back) recruitment when doing pull-ups. Obviously, this is better for getting a bigger, wider back.

- Once you get good at pull-ups, start doing static holds for one second.

Static holds are awesome for getting your back really wide, fast. But they're hard, so you have to be careful with when you do them. First master pull-ups. Once you can do 10 or more pull-ups, then you can start incorporating static holds into your pull-up sets.

Static holds simply require stopping about halfway down after completing a pull-up and holding yourself in place for one second. You pause and hold in that spot on your way down. Then after you do the one-second pause, you go down until your arms are locked out.

Again, since you'll be using the Effortless Exercise System while doing pull-ups, this means you'll never go to failure. So if you can do a maximum of say 10 pull-ups, you'll only be doing sets of 3 to 5 reps of pull-ups.

Note: The best time to do static holds is after you complete the last rep of each set.

Also, the key to doing static holds is to feel the tension in your lats (your latissimus dorsi muscles), not in your biceps or forearms.

To give you an idea on how powerful doing low rep pull-ups are, I built up to doing 28 pull-ups on a max set simply by doing a lot of 3 to 6 rep sets of pull-ups. I'll talk about this more in a little bit, but for pull-ups you will need to work up to doing 50 to 100 a day, six days a week.

Don't worry, I'll soon show you how to squeeze that into a busy schedule.

Burpees

Burpees will be the focus of this section. Burpees comprise the primary exercise that convicts use to get bigger, stronger, more ripped, and build athleticism into their bodies. Getting bigger and stronger don't mean anything if you don't know how to move your body in a fight.

Here's how to do burpees:

1. Begin in a squat position with your hands on the floor in front of you.

2. Kick your feet back while you go down into a pushup.

3. As you're pushing up with the pushup, return your feet into the previous squat position.

4. Jump up as high as you can from the squat position.

5. Keep repeating, doing them as fast as possible.

These are harder than pushups. In my opinion, burpees are *better* than pushups too.

Not only will you get a bigger chest from doing these, but you'll get ripped up (fast) and get in great condition while gaining muscle mass all over your body. There's a reason why prisoners do them: they work and they do so much for you beyond simply getting bigger, stronger, and a better looking chest.

I don't know you or your conditioning or your athletic ability, but definitely try to incorporate these into your workouts.

Of course, following the Effortless Exercise System's rules, you don't do burpees to failure. If you can do 10 total burpees until failure (test yourself to see your maximum), then you'd end up doing sets of 3 to 5 reps. Again, somewhere between 30 to 50% of your best set.

To illustrate the proper way to do these, I did a quick Google search so you can see a video and picture of how to do them.

Here's a picture of burpees:

http://myfitnesshut.blogspot.com/2010/11/burpees-burn-fat.html

Here's a video of burpees:

http://www.youtube.com/watch?v=c_Dq_NCzj8M

> **Note:** Pushups, pull-ups, and burpees are the three main exercises I want you to put your focus on if you can. Those will get the most bang for your buck within the Effortless Exercise System rules.

With the *big three* out of the way, what follows are some other exercises you can throw into your workouts as well.

Hindu Squats

Hindu squats are awesome for building explosive muscular endurance. If you're an athlete or want to build athleticism into your body – the type of athleticism where you keep going and going and going – do Hindu squats.

> **Note:** Barbell squats for most people are more trouble than they're worth. They're not necessary and they cause too much stress to your body. They're great for strength and gaining mass all over your body, but a lot of people don't really benefit from them. If you like doing barbell squats, then by all means, keep doing them. Simply use the Effortless Exercise System principles while doing them and you'll get bigger, stronger, and more explosive.

I personally prefer Hindu Squats over barbell squats because I can do them at home at my convenience.

Hindu Squats *are not* normal bodyweight squats where you go up and down. Hindu Squats instead have more rhythm to them. One of the most important things about Hindu Squats is you inhale on the way up and exhale on the way down. It's the opposite of normal squatting. Make sure to take deep breaths in order to improve the power of your lungs.

So keep a rhythm both with the actual squatting and with your breathing.

Here is a picture and video of Hindu Squats I found doing a quick Google search:

http://extremebodyweightworkouts.com/blog/hindu-squats-harder-than-they-look

Let me point out something about the video. If possible, I want you to swipe your fingertips against the ground while doing Hindu Squats. In the video the guy didn't bring his arms down far enough in my opinion.

You can do these to the point of sweating if you want and use them as a cardio workout. That's fine. But I prefer that you use them within the guidelines of the Effortless Exercise System. This means of course you are not going anywhere near failure and you're not doing too many reps.

It's up to you how you approach it of course.

Later, I'll give you some examples of how to incorporate them into workouts.

Stair Runs/Walks

Okay, this is one exercise where you won't be following my Effortless Exercise System. There are always exceptions that help prove the rule. This is one of them.

Effortless Exercise System for Men

Stair Runs/Walks are awesome for burning off fat and getting ripped. But doing them can be extremely intense. If you have stairs in your home or close by; awesome. This will make doing these very convenient. They only take five minutes of your time.

What you do is run up one to three flights of stairs and walk back down. Keep repeating that *non-stop* (that's key) for five minutes. You'll get your rests on the walks down the stairs. As you can determine, this forms an active rest and not a passive rest.

That's it. Run up the stairs. Walk back down.

If you need help building up to doing the full five minutes non-stop, then periodically mix in a few walks up the stairs instead of doing the runs. If you're way out of shape, just start with walking both up and down the stairs and then mix in some runs up the stairs. As you build up, if your goal is to get as ripped up as possible and get 6-pack abs, then do this five to six days a week.

Once you're doing the full five minutes non-stop as outlined, you'll see results in the mirror sometime in the second week. They're fast-acting. You *don't* need any other type of cardio if you do these stair runs/walks. So just 25 to 30 minutes of total cardio for the week.

I can't recommend these enough. And by the way, you actually can *sort of* use the Effortless Exercise System principles to do these exercises as well. Let's say you have stairs at home. Just run up them and walk back down. Do that every once in a while. If you could get in a total of 20 sets of doing that, you'll be good to go.

In fact, that's a great way to build up to being able to do five minutes of them when you first begin.

Biceps Curls

Hopefully you have some adjustable weight dumbbells at home. If not, go get some. If you don't do that, then you can't do these exercises the way I'm going to outline them for you.

> **Note:** Believe me, I'm not going to keep suggesting that you purchase equipment and spend a fortune. Only a few things are necessary for superior muscle growth and fat loss and physique.

One of the best things you can do to grow your arms is to do one set of curls once an hour, all day. Follow each biceps curl set with one set of pushups with your hands close together (within six inches of touching) so the emphasis is on your triceps and not your chest. Whatever your 10 rep maximum weight is for dumbbells, only do 6 reps. That's it; no more, no less.

Do a set of six reps for biceps curls every hour followed by a set of 6 to 10 pushups. If you did that three times a week, you'll gain *at least* one inch in your arms within one month. *Guaranteed!*

Another way to accomplish the same results without having to "fit it into your day" is to follow this routine is using mini-workouts or, even better, during TV commercials.

Think about that. You can gain an inch in your arms in one month *without* sweating. These principles are powerful stuff. Put it all to the test and prove me wrong. I dare you. By the way, I'll expand on this for gaining arm size in one of the bonus reports.

Swings

These offer another great way to burn off fat and get ripped up. Buy a kettlebell or build yourself a t-bar for swings.

Here's a video I found doing a quick Google search:

http://www.youtube.com/watch?v=0_XjJjLc7NE

You can do swings for time or by reps.

If you do them for reps, use the Effortless Exercise System's rules. Determine the maximum amount of reps you can do until failure and then do 30 to 50% of those reps per set. This means if you can do 20 total swings in a set, then you'd end up doing 6 to 10 per set. When beginning, I always urge people to stick closer to the 30%.

Remember, the Effortless Exercise System is all about making exercising easy and never making it hard. Exercise doesn't need to be hard for you to get stronger and bigger. That's a myth that does nothing but cause us to quit before we see decent results.

Jumping Jacks

Let's be clear – You won't get bigger or stronger doing jumping jacks.

So why did I include them? Because jumping jacks are actually a great conditioning exercise if you follow one simple rule in doing them. That rule is this: perform the jumping jacks as fast and *explosively* as possible.

Again, using the Effortless Exercise System rules, do 30 to 50% of your maximum for sets. This means, if you can normally do 30 jumping jacks in a row until you can't do any more, you instead do 9 to 15 explosive, fast jumping jacks per set. For me, I never go above 10. I simply do 10 per set.

This exercise is more a throw-in that is wonderful for an overall body conditioner.

If you don't do them as fast as possible and as explosively as possible, don't even bother with the jumping jacks. Just in case you want to see how to do jumping jacks, here is a quick video I found through a Google search:

http://www.youtube.com/watch?v=dmYwZH_BNd0

> **Note:** In the video, he did *not* do the jumping jacks explosively or as fast as possible. You however should.

Bear Crawls

Bear crawls are awesome for your entire body. In fact, I heavily use this exercise while training my 3-year old son (he's now 5 and a half as I write this). Here's some quick inspiration for you. I practice what I preach in this book with my son. Before he even turned 5 years old, he could do 14 consecutive pull-ups, non-stop... *and*, that was with less than one year of training pull-ups. Need I say more?

Back to bear crawls. It's just as you suspected. You do the bear crawl by mimicking how a bear walks. So you'll be walking with both your feet and hands. This truly strengthens your shoulders and arms.

If you didn't realize it, farmers are some of the naturally strongest people you'll ever meet. It's because of the routine tasks they must do often on the farm. Such movement builds functional, non-weight room strength into their bodies. That's why I love bodyweight exercises. They build strength you can use out in the real world.

Not all of your weight room strength will transfer out into the real world. A lot of times guys who are strong in the gym are weak at doing typical guy things out of the gym. I was just using farmers as an example. No, they don't do bear crawls. But bear crawls, just as the movements farmers use, will enable you to perform better if you have a physical job or play sports.

Bear crawls are one of the most unique and interesting bodyweight exercises that work to strengthen your entire body. As a bonus, they are great for basic cardio too. For my son, I simply have him do 15 feet of bear crawls back and forth in our living room. He loves them!

He can do up to a quarter mile of bear crawls in a single day and not be sore the next day. He's going to be a beast when he gets older. Again, he was doing this at the age of three. So if he does and loves them, what is *your* excuse? Do I need to bribe you with cookies and lollipops as I used to do with my son?

There really isn't a way to implement the Effortless Exercise System principles with bear crawls. Just don't do the exercise to the point of getting tired or sweating.

Below is a video I found with a Google search of bear crawls. Although the woman shows you how to do them backwards and sideways, those aren't needed. Just do them going forward.

http://www.youtube.com/watch?v=udIpJF4ZDY0

BONUS SECTION!
JACKED: HOW CONVICTS IN PRISON GET JACKED UP FAST

Most people think convicts get big and strong in prison from doing a ton of weightlifting.

Actually, that's not the case.

Most prisons removed weights decades ago. They didn't want prisoners to use weights in prisons as a sort of breeding ground to get bigger and stronger. Such would make them more physically dominant when they got out.

With limited space and limited (or no) equipment, prisoners had to figure out what to do to get bigger and stronger than other prisoners for their mere survival in prison. Prisoners aren't totally stupid. They switched to bodyweight exercises and are just as jacked up; and possibly more so than before.

Their main exercise is the burpee. They need functional strength and athleticism in order to survive in prison. The burpee gives that to them. I told you about the burpee earlier and gave you links on how to do them so I won't get into the details of here.

Effortless Exercise System for Men

Here, I'm going to tell you how convicts do their burpee workouts. Then I'll tell you how to do them using Effortless Exercise System principles. You can choose to do them however you want.

If you want to be totally hardcore about burpees like guys in prison, do it the way they do them. You may see even better results if you do, but the problem with that is you'll be sweating and it'll be hard to do them. This means you'll probably have a hard time doing them daily.

With my preferred way, you can do a lot of burpees without sweating, without them being hard, and you can do a lot of sets and reps daily without a problem. Anyway, prisoners do reverse pyramid, descending sets with burpees.

To do burpees the prisoner way, start with doing 20 burpees. 20 burpees are quite hard for a beginner (heck, they aren't easy even for people who do burpees often). If you've never done burpees before or are out of shape, you'll need to work up to 20. 20 make a full set. If they're doing these in their cell, they rest 10 to 30 seconds and then do 19 burpees for the next set. If they're in the yard, they just walk to the other end of the yard using those 10 to 30 seconds as a walking rest and then do the next set.

They continue doing descending sets: 18, 17, 16, 15, 14, and so on down to one using 10 to 30 second rests. This means they get in a total of 210 burpees in 15 minutes or less. That is quite a challenge.

If that's too hard for you to do (assume it is), start with doing 10 descending sets in that manner (for a total of 55 burpees).

Then build up to 20. In prison, if you can't do 20 descending scts starting with 20 burpees, you're not considered a man.

If you want to be considered a "stud" in prison, you need to be able to do 30 descending sets starting with 30 burpees down to one. That's a total of 465 burpees!

You can do that if you want, but that's plain hard. Plus, hopefully you're not in prison so it's probably not a life or death struggle for survival and respect that you work up to 30 descending sets.

I prefer – and I suspect most of my readers will prefer to go the Effortless Exercise System route. For that, it's simple. Just determine the maximum amount of burpees you can do for a set. Let's say it is 15 to 20 burpees. What you want to do are sets of 5 to 10 burpees with a 30-45 second rest between them. Do as many sets as it takes to do 100 burpees in a day. You can do them all in a row and it'll take you 10 to 15 minutes (you'll end up sweating if you do it this way). Or you can do a set every once in a while during the day until you do 100 total burpees.

However you fit them in doesn't matter. Just do the 100 total burpees each day.

Now, if you're already doing 100 pushups a day, you may not want to do 100 total burpees a day too, since burpees also incorporate a pushup. Remember, burpees are harder than pushups and overall, burpees are better for your core. So if you had to choose between doing either of them, I'd encourage you to do burpees.

But it's your choice. Both are great and can be done together or separately. Either way, if you did 100 burpees a day or 100 pushups a day for a month, your chest will be way bigger. *Guaranteed.*

If you did 100 of both of them each day (for most guys that's simply too much), your chest and whole body would be bigger, stronger, and more athletic in 30 days. If you only had a few pounds to lose when you started, you'd also be ultra-ripped by day 30 of doing both.

Don't believe me? Do it and prove me wrong. Whatever it takes to get you to do it, I'm all for. If I have to challenge you, so be it. And in 30 days, you'll be 30 days older either way. The 30th day is coming barring some misfortune. So at Day 30 you would have done them and improved your body beyond belief or you can still be deciding if you should.

Just please use my system and do these exercises. 30 days. One month. You'll be glad you did. I promise.

These things are simple and the workouts are fairly easy to do, but they're powerful and they get fast results. If you are anything like I was, you thought weights were the be-all, end-all as far as working out.

Years ago back in college I bench pressed 435 pounds. But my chest right now is bigger than it was back then. I thank burpees and pushups. I'm in my mid-30's now and I haven't bench pressed in over four years. The last time I remember bench pressing I did 150 pound dumbbells (so 300 pounds) for eight reps. That amount translates to around a 400 pound bench press (let's say 405 to make it a nice 4 plates on each side).

But still, my chest is better *now* than it was doing dumbbell bench presses. Sure, I probably have a weak bench press now compared to those numbers. Although pushups and burpees do help translate into strength in the bench press, it's still not the same as doing the bench press to get stronger in the bench press.

Remember: the *specificity* part of superior performance.

> **Note:** I also squatted 500 pounds for 10 reps in college. But even doing that, my legs weren't big. Four years ago I also stopped squatting. I instead started to focus on Hindu Squats. My legs are now bigger and look better than when I squatted 500 for ten reps. As I got older, I realized that I was lifting more for my ego than anything else. Once I dropped my ego and put more focus on the bodyweight exercises described here in this book, my body got better and my functional (real world) strength also got better.

I still love weightlifting and do it, don't get me wrong. And in a future book, I'll probably talk about how I do my weightlifting these days. But the point I'm trying to make to you is to simply keep an open mind and don't think it's either or in regards to bodyweight exercises vs. weightlifting.

Again, as I mentioned earlier, you can use the Effortless Exercise System principles for weightlifting as well. And if you do so, you will see *awesome* results.

Back to convicts. They mostly focus on burpees. But they also like to do pull-ups and pushups too. With pushups and pull-ups, they simply use a lot of volume. This translates to lots of sets, lots of reps, and short rest times. The only major difference from the Effortless Exercise System is that convicts do a lot of reps per set whereas I advise you to do a lower amount of reps per set.

Regardless, you can take away something from prisoners and how they work out. They get bigger, stronger, and more ripped with minimal equipment while eating crappy prison food that doesn't have enough calories or protein in it.

You'll see a similar pattern to successfully getting bigger, stronger, and ripped without weights in the next section about Herschel Walker.

What *You* Can Learn from Herschel Walker's Workouts

Just in case you don't know who Herschel Walker is, I'll give you a quick rundown. He was the Heisman Award winner (best college football player) in 1982 playing running back for the University of Georgia. Then he played professional football from 1983 to 1997. But who cares about all that?

What concerns us here is that he is 225 pounds of ripped muscle at the age of 53. And he even started doing professional MMA in 2009 at the age of 47. So far, he's 2 and 0 in MMA and still fighting.

How is he able to do all of this at his age?

Besides being a gifted and dedicated athlete, he specifically does bodyweight exercises to stay in shape.

He does an insane amount of volume.

He does 1,000+ pushups daily.

He also does 3,500 sit-ups daily.

> **Note:** Don't do sit-ups. They suck and they're bad for your back. I'm just telling you what he does. Not everything he does is useful. In the case of sit-ups, he's wasting his time. Remember, when he started doing these bodyweight routines, it was in the late 1970's and they simply didn't know what we know today about sit-ups. If you're going to do anything, do crunches and only go 1/4 to 1/3 the way up to keep the focus on your abs and save yourself from back problems.

I'm not sure if he still does these, but he has also done 1,500 pull-ups and 1,000 dips a day too. Now that's impressive.

But honestly, all that isn't needed. It's overkill. If you're like me, you don't want to spend your whole day working out to get in all those sets and reps. He mentioned doing these exercises during TV commercials (and that leads me into the next chapter on how I do most of my exercising), but still, to fit in all that volume goes beyond just working out during TV commercials.

You're busy, I'm busy. Hershel Walker's exercise volume won't be happening for us. All that working out is a great attribute to his dedication, but it's not efficient or smart in my opinion. The reason why I added this section to the book is to reinforce the idea that bodyweight exercises are truly all you need. Or at the very least, they can be a big part of your workouts.

I don't think convicts or Herschel Walker use bodyweight exercises efficiently, but there's no denying the awesome results they get from doing them. By the way, here's a link to an article that has a picture of Herschel Walker at 48 and also a short video clip of him talking about his workouts. Seriously, look at that picture of him and keep reminding yourself that he's 48 and only does bodyweight exercises!

http://www.tryingfitness.com/herschel-walker-workout/

TV COMMERCIAL WORKOUTS & MINI-WORKOUTS

If you didn't watch that video clip of Herschel Walker above, he mentioned that he used to (and maybe still does) workout during TV commercials. Although I've been doing this long before I read that he does it, it just reinforces my thinking on the subject.

Short mini-workouts of 2 to 10 minutes are the way to go to get bigger, stronger, and more ripped. I use a combination of working out during 2 to 3 minute TV commercials and doing 5 to 10 minute mini-workouts.

The primary reason why the Effortless Exercise System is so successful at transforming a person's body is because it sticks to the principle of "doing as much quality exercise as possible while staying as fresh as possible."

You can definitely work the Effortless Exercise System into long workouts if you want. They work great for that. But I strongly recommend sticking with doing multiple 2 to 10 minute mini-workouts daily. If you watch a lot of TV or are on your computer a lot, these mini-workouts fit in perfectly. A one-hour TV show has around eight commercial breaks of about 2.5 minutes each for a total of 20 minutes you can fit in your working out.

If you were to watch just one hour of TV like this, you can get in 20 minutes of working out. If you watch more than an hour of TV with commercials, you can get even more working out done. Throw in a few hours at your computer; where you can get up every 5 to 10 minutes and do a quick set of pushups, burpees, Hindu Squats, or pull-ups.

That's a lot of working out you could easily fit into your day.

And none of this working out would make you sweat. None of it would be physically hard for you. And it doesn't really interfere with your life. And your Nervous System isn't stretched to capacity.

Doing so many means you're just using wasted time (TV commercials) and downtime (while you're on the computer).

GIVE ME 30

So, can you give the Effortless Exercise System a try for 30 days?

If you give me just 30 days, you'll literally start to transform your body. After 30 days, you can adjust the system to suit yourself better. You won't have to do these workouts every day if you don't want to. I just want you to do them for 30 days in a row the first month to prove that this way of working out works for you.

I want you to have the confidence in knowing that you'll never need to work out at a gym again if you don't want to. I want you to be confident that you can have a nice body without sweating, without struggling through sets, and without having to waste time in a busy schedule.

If all you can spare is 20 minutes of TV commercials once a day during just one hour of TV time, that's fine. You'll get awesome results from that alone. If you can do more commercial break mini-workouts, do more. If you can fit in a quick 10 minute mini-workout early in the day and another 10 minute mini-workout later at night (in addition to the TV commercial workouts), that's even better.

Play around with how you do this; however you want. Just understand that it's flexible and it's your choice how you want to time your workouts and which exercises you want to use. The main thing is you follow the core rules to the system.

Avoid fatigue. Stay fresh while working out. This means not going to muscular failure during an exercise. Never struggle doing a set. All sets should be relatively easy.

Do a lot of sets, but make sure the reps per set are low.

Keep your rest times short so you can fit in more sets. Since you're not going to muscular failure, you don't need long rest times since you're staying fresh. Be sure to do a lot of little workouts instead of one big workout. Make sure the exercises are challenging you.

The exercises should be moderately hard and you'll do them intensely, but the actual sets will be easy because again, you aren't going to failure during any set. Let the total volume take care of you getting bigger and stronger. Each individual set is meaningless except for what it contributes to the whole of the volume.

SAMPLE WORKOUT GUIDES AND ROUTINE OUTLINES

Here are some sample workouts you can use. If you want to modify them to suit your work and lifestyle, feel free. Use them as a guide to create your own workouts. As long as you follow the key concepts, have fun creating your own workouts. Try new things. See what works and what doesn't.

In all honesty, the workouts aren't anything special in my opinion. They get the job done, but they're nothing special. The only reason they are special resides in the key concepts and principles you're following in the Effortless Exercise System.

That's where the magic is.

Prepping for the Routines

First, before you do any exercise, figure out how many reps you can do for a maximum set. You need to do this to determine the correct amount of reps to do per set in order to make each set easy. So test out how many pushups you can do for a set. Same with pull-ups, burpees, Hindu Squats, and so on. This is the only time I want you to go to muscular failure.

For biceps curls, determine the weight you can use for 10 to 12 reps using dumbbells. That'll be the weight you use for your sets of curls. You'll do 6 to 7 reps for each set of curls.

Note: For curls, I prefer to go up to 60 to 70% of my maximum. The reason you can do this is because the bicep is a relatively small muscle and doesn't have much of an effect on your Nervous System.

Once you figure out how many you can do, remember that each set you do will have to be around 30 to 50% of the total reps you did to failure.

But that is only a general rule. If necessary, you can go below the 30% level. I'm able to do 28 pull-ups for my max set. But I *never* go above 5 to 6 pull-ups in a set. That's less than a 20% level. Just know you can play around with this. You need to make sure the set is easy to do and that the following set will also be easy to do. You don't want to accumulate fatigue and make your following sets harder.

Anyway, say you did 20 pushups for a max set. That means you'll be doing sets of 6 to 10 reps. Take note that when you begin doing this system, stick closer to doing reps at the 30% level of a max set and work from there.

In the above case with 20 pushups, I want you to start doing sets of 6 pushups.

As you get used to doing these, you can try and tick the number of reps per set up while staying within the guidelines. You'll usually find a "sweet spot" that you like and just stick with that until you've gotten so strong you need to progress past it.

Here's your goal: 100 pushup daily.

What I do personally is 10 to 15 sets of 6 to 10 pushups for a total of 100 pushups. Remember to do the pushups as I outlined above. Don't do pushups the way everyone else does them. Those mostly work your triceps, not your chest.

I just do pushups and not the advanced feet-elevated pushups or clap pushups. That's a personal preference for me because I like to focus more on burpees rather than pushups. I like the added dimension of the burpees also being an athletic, total body movement.

For pull-ups, your goal is 50 to 100 a day. Remember this. Out of all the exercises listed, pull-ups are the most neurologically demanding exercise. That's why even though I can do 28 pull-ups, I only do sets of 5 to 6 pull-ups. It's too easy to burn out your Nervous System with pull-ups. The most pull-ups I ever did were 200 in 22 to 23 minutes. I did 40 sets of 5 reps with about 30 seconds rest between sets.

Now as you can see, I sort of broke my rule of short 2 to 10 minute workouts.

But as I've mentioned a few times, you can use the Effortless Exercise System rules within normal workouts. That's fine. Just stick to the rules and you'll be fine.

My normal pull-ups workout (when I'm strictly doing only pull-ups and not jumping between sets of pull-ups, burpees, and pushups) is to do 20 sets of 5 reps. I do these during TV commercials. I'm able to squeeze in about 5 sets of 5 reps for each commercial break. So it takes me four commercial breaks to do 100 reps of pull-ups. That equates to about 30 minutes of watching TV.

For burpees, your goal is 100 burpees a day.

On the pushup part of burpees, I'm not strict as I am on pushups. I'm not thinking about pulling my hands in together or squeezing my chest together, or locking out my arms as far as possible. I normally do 10 sets of 10 reps of burpees.

If I'm doing them during TV commercials, I normally do 3 to 4 sets for each 2 and a half minute commercial. I rest 30 seconds between sets usually.

Those are my big 3 exercises: burpees, pushups, and pull-ups.

Everything else, although good, I consider for myself (you may be different) an afterthought.

I'm not as strict with the following routines. I do them, but I don't do them daily and if I miss doing them, it's not a big deal as long as I'm consistently doing the 3 big exercises.

For Hindu Squats, I normally do sets of 15. I don't even know my max set of Hindu Squats. If your goal is more to get ripped and bring out your abs as best as possible, you may want to put more focus on doing Hindu Squats.

I usually mix them in once every so often when I'm doing my jump sets workout where I start with 10 burpees, then do 5 pull-ups, and then do 6 push-ups.

> **Note:** Just so you know, when I do mixed workouts like that and I'm jumping between different exercises, my rest times are shorter.

In fact, a lot of times I don't even rest until after the third set. The reason I do that and the reason I'm able to get away with that and stay fresh is due to the order of my exercises. Burpees are a total body exercise, but they don't put much stress on your upper back. So my back is relatively fresh to do the pull-ups. So, I do those immediately after the burpees.

Because the pull-ups work the back and not the chest, my chest is getting a little bit of a rest while doing the pull-ups. That means once I'm done with the pull-ups, I can do pushups right away without a rest. Then after I'm done with the pushups, I take a 30 second rest and repeat that sequence.

I can get three of those sequences in each TV commercial break. This means three sets of burpees, three sets of pull-ups, and three sets of pushups.

That's my main way of working out because I can get a lot of sets done in very little time.

> **Note:** I do have a pull-up station at home and I suggest you get one. But if you just can't because of money or space, don't worry too much about it. If you go to the gym, you can use the Effortless Exercise System principles to do a quick 50 pull-ups. In fact, I'll tell you right now how I do pull-ups at the gym. I do my normal workout and between every couple of sets while I'm resting, I do five pull-ups. Sometimes I simply do jump sets where I do whatever exercise I'm doing and then immediately do a set of pull-ups right after. I continue doing that until I've done my 50 total pull-ups.

Okay, back to Hindu Squats. I do sets of 15 of those. Mostly during the week I put very little focus on doing them, although I throw them in once in a while here and there. But usually once a week I put more focus on Hindu Squats. And on that day, I'll do 150 total Hindu Squats. I do this by doing 10 sets of 15. Now, that's just me. Use the system however you want since no two people have the same exact goals or abilities.

For stair runs, I usually do these once or twice a week. These are brutal when doing them for five minutes non-stop. Anything more than twice a week and it sometimes affects the rest of my working out. But if I ever want to rip up more and get totally shredded and cut, I'd cut back on the burpees, pushups, and pull-ups and do these stair runs once or twice a day for 5 to 6 days a week for 2 weeks.

In two weeks, your abs will look ridiculous. It's unbelievable how effective these stair runs/walks are for melting fat off your belly. Then after two weeks, I go back to doing my normal workouts. Remember, you can also do the stair runs/walks using my Effortless Exercise System rules by doing something like one stair run at a time.

So you run up 1 to 3 flights of stairs and walk back down. Then you're done. Then you do it again 30 minutes, 1 hour, or 2 hours later. Or you can do 1 to 2 stair run/walks per TV commercial if you have stairs in your home.

I personally don't use my Effortless Exercise System rules for stair runs/walks. But I think they're perfect for people who are out of shape and want to eventually do the full five minutes of stair runs/walks.

For swings, I do 10 to 15 swings at a time using a 40 to 50 pound t-bar that I created to replace having to get multiple kettlebells. As with Hindu Squats, I don't put much focus on doing swings. They're great, don't get me wrong. But hey, we each have our preferences... and for simplicity's sake, it's best not to do too many different exercises daily.

I still do swing often, usually at least one set a day. It's just hard for me to break into my routine using the big 3 exercises. As with Hindu Squats, I also like to put the focus on swings about once a week. In that case, I normally do 10 sets of 15 swings.

Now on to Bear Crawls… I love them!

The only problem is I don't have enough space in my home to do them the way I want to do them. A small space is okay for my son to do them; 15 feet going back and forth in my living room. But for me, I prefer to do these 50 feet each time I do them.

For that, I need to do them outside.

I've gotten so spoiled by my easy, indoor Effortless Exercise System workouts that I don't like having to be inconvenienced into going outside to do workouts. Once you start doing this, you'll see what I mean. So honestly, I'm just too lazy to do these much. And yes, I still see great results week after week, year after year.

I'm content watching my son do them. Plus I live in Texas. Six months out of the year it's in the 90's or 100's. So forget going outside to work out. When I do in fact do bear crawls, I like to do 10 bear crawls of 50 feet for a total of 500 feet. I rest one minute between sets.

About Jumping Jacks... I always thought these were stupid until I learned how important it was to do them as fast as possible while being as explosive as possible. I use them a lot as filler in my burpees/pushups/pull-ups workouts. I try to get 10 sets of 10 Jumping Jacks done every day. But unlike burpees, pushups, and pull-ups, I'm not as strict and hardcore about getting all that work in each day.

If I do it great; that's my goal. But if I don't do them it isn't a big deal. Remember, this is just me. You need to take these principles and do what you want.

I will say this about Jumping Jacks: *Wow*. Your arms get really fast and explosive doing these. Your legs get really fast too. If you want to build athleticism into your body, doing these with burpees is a great combination.

For biceps curls, if you want to gain at least one inch to your arms in less than a month, pay attention to how I do these! A lot of people actually have gained a half inch in just *one day* doing them! (Myself included.)

This goes beyond what I mentioned above for getting bigger arms.

First figure out what your 10 to 12 rep maximum weight is using dumbbells. With that weight, you'll do sets of 6 to 7 reps. You're going to need to do this at home and you'll need to do it when you're not busy and have the whole day. For most people, a weekend day would work.

In fact, here's an idea I just got as I'm writing this. It's not football season right now, but you can do this biceps routine on a Sunday and watch football all day. If not football, just watch TV all day. Make sure whatever you're watching has commercials.

I recommend that you don't do any other exercises also. Skip doing burpees, pushups, pull-ups, and everything else.

Just do curls and follow them up with a set of pushups with your hands close together.

And let me be clear here, the next day you're probably going to feel these, and that's probably an understatement. What you do is two sets of curls (6 to 7 reps) during each TV commercial break. Do the curls fast. Don't use a slow tempo. In fact, no matter what exercise you do, do it fast.

After one set of curls, immediately do a set of 6 to 7 pushups with your hands close together; like a triangle (note that these pushups are different than the pushups you do to build up your chest). Then rest about 45 seconds before doing the next two sets (One set of curls and one of pushups).

Stay with me, we're almost done.

Now do a total of 50 sets of curls and 50 sets of pushups for the day. You can do them every single commercial break (I don't recommend that) or you can skip commercial breaks. Doesn't matter. Just do a total of 50 sets for each exercise in 9 hours or less.

I recommend you do this once a week for 4 weeks in order to gain at least an inch in your arms. After that, do this just once every few months since the gains aren't as drastic after you've done this routine the initial four times in 1 month. I either do two sets of each exercise every other commercial break or I do two sets during one commercial break and one set the following commercial break. I follow that pattern until I've done 50 sets of both curls and pushups.

Make sure to have a piece of paper nearby and mark off the sets as you do them.

I write the numbers 1 to 50 on a piece of paper and X them out as I do the sets. This workout is simple... but it's not easy. The results are worth it.

An easier, but less dramatic, way to get bigger arms is to add in some curls during your normal TV commercial workouts or mini-workouts while also doing your other exercises. A routine I use a lot is to do a set of either burpees or pushups followed by a set of pull-ups, and then a set of curls. I do that sequence 2 to 3 times during a commercial break.

If you don't have adjustable weight dumbbells, hopefully you'll get some and start incorporating curls using the above as an outline.

Remember, this is just a more concentrated version than I talked about earlier in this book. Doing it this way, you'll only need to do work your arms like this once a week.

The other way is daily and with less volume.

WHAT TO DO IF YOU HIT A PLATEAU

We all hit plateaus. Our bodies come to a standstill, right when we are seeing great results. So what do you do if you hit a plateau where your workouts just don't feel like they're getting any results and where you feel more tired and less motivated to work out?

If you're using the Effortless Exercise System correctly, this shouldn't happen to any great extent. Sure, there'll be times when you can't fit in the workout. That happens. Although I recommend you do these workouts daily (and I insist you do them daily for the first 30 days), you don't have to do them every day.

But the way they're set up with the TV commercial workouts and other mini-workouts, why not do these every day? They're easy. These workouts will separate you from all the other guys out there.

Your body will be one of the elites in society. People will notice that. Trust me on this. You get a lot of respect by having a nice body.

Anyway, when and if it ever comes down to you hitting a plateau or you don't feel motivated to do these workouts often, then the main thing you have to do is cut back the amount of sets you do, cut back the amount of reps you do for each set, increase your rest times, and take 1 or 2 extra days off for 1 or 2 weeks.

That should do the trick. Make your individual sets and your workouts even easier than they already were. Truly, this is an effortless system. If it feels like effort to you, then you need to cut back and make it so it doesn't feel like an effort.

You should also take a serious look at you training and maybe make some changes to it (besides the cutting back). Remember, no set should ever feel like it took a lot of effort. Each set should be a challenge, but it still should be easy and effortless.

When you hit a plateau, cut back and make things easier. Then after 1 to 2 weeks, start adding back reps and sets while shortening up your rest times.

Note: Bad nutrition, lack of sleep, and stress also contribute to plateaus.

FAQ – FREQUENTLY ASKED QUESTIONS

After teaching and training and writing about the Effortless Exercise System for years, I get a lot of questions. Several overlap and frequently come up. I want to take a few minutes to address the more common questions and give you answers so you aren't left wondering about some sideline issues.

Q: Do I have to do the exercises you listed?

A: No, those are just examples. But they're highly effective exercises.

I personally use them and I know my system works effectively with them to get incredible results. Thousands of people have gotten strength results as well as body composition results using the principles of the Effortless Exercise System while getting more ripped.

You can use the Effortless Exercise System rules for most weightlifting exercises. I don't weightlift as often as I used to since all I really need to make and keep my body looking awesome is to do burpees, pushups, and pull-ups, but I still use these rules while weightlifting. At my best while weightlifting, I weighed 242 pounds at about 8% body fat. That was when I was in college years ago.

Now, with a wife and two little boys and being in my mid 30's, I'm 226 pounds at about 9% body fat. I'm still strong and I look great. In fact, although I was bigger at 242 pounds, my body actually looks nicer now at 226 pounds even though I'm more than ten years older. The reason I look better is because of the exercises I listed in this book. They're simply more effective for making your body look nicer.

Sure, you'll probably be stronger lifting weights, but I'm still stronger than almost all people who lift weights even though I rarely lift weights these days. And to be honest, if I wanted to gain more muscle and get up to the 240 pound range again, I wouldn't even need to weightlift. I'd still do the same bodyweight exercises. The only thing I'd change is how I ate. I'd eat more calories to gain the extra muscle.

To make sure I didn't gain fat, I'd simply increase the amounts of sets I did each day for my bodyweight exercises. It's not all about using weights to gain muscle.

And if I wanted to get more ripped up and down to the 7-8% body fat range, I'd just tighten up my diet a little and do the stair runs/walks once or twice a day for 2 weeks.

Q: Are you saying your way is the only way to get bigger and stronger?

A: No, definitely not.

There are a lot of ways to get bigger and stronger. My system is just the simplest, the easiest, and the most convenient way. Look, you're not going to become a top ranked power lifter or Olympic lifter using the exercises I listed. To get good at powerlifting or Olympic lifting, you have to do them. It's the specificity rule.

But, having said that, a lot of powerlifters and Olympic lifters use the same core rules as I outlined here. They don't use them exactly as I do, but they do use them.

If you don't want to go full-fledge into doing my system, you don't have to. Use the key rules I outline as a guide and start to incorporate them into how you exercise. Whatever results you're getting now will improve by adding some of my rules in.

Q: How many days a week do I need to do this?

A: You can use this system however many days you want each week. If you're using the bodyweight exercises I recommend, I suggest you do this 5 to 6 days a week. If possible, do these every day for the first month.

If you're doing this as outlined in mini-workouts and during TV commercials... that should be simple to manage even if you're extremely busy. If you use the Effortless Exercise System for weightlifting, use it each time you weightlift. You'll get stronger and bigger a lot faster if you do.

Q: How long do I have to exercise each day using this method?

A: 20 minutes minimum a day is ideal.

Depending on your level, it may be more important to instead use total reps as guidelines instead of minutes. Ideally, you'd do 100 pushups, 100 burpees, and 50 to 100 pull-ups a day while throwing in some of the other exercises as well.

But, your goals may be radically different from mine. If you want a bigger chest, focus on burpees and pushups. If you want a bigger, wider back, focus on doing pull-ups. If you want better legs, focus on doing Hindu Squats and stair runs/walks. Bigger arms? Curls and triangle pushups with your hands close together. For athletic movement you want to do burpees, bear crawls, and explosive Jumping Jacks.

To lose fat, focus on stair runs/walks, burpees, bear crawls, swings, and Hindu squats.

You can also concentrate on one different exercise a day.

For example, this routine is a good one for a daily exercise schedule:

- Mondays… burpees

- Tuesdays… pull-ups

- Wednesdays… pushups

- Thursdays… Hindu squats

- Fridays… bear crawls and swings

- Saturdays… curls

- Sunday… off

It's totally up to you. What you do depends on your goals and how fast you want to achieve them and also how dedicated you are to improving yourself physically.

Q: What if I can only do a few reps as my max for an exercise?

A: If you can only do a few reps of an exercise, then you'll need to start by doing sets of one rep to build up your strength. Don't worry. A lot of people have to start right here.

For exercises like burpees and pushups, instead of having a goal of 100 reps for the day, shoot for a goal of 25 to 35 sets of one rep. Your strength will build up fast by doing this.

For an exercise like pull-ups, again, do sets of one pull-up and shoot for say 20 total reps in a day. A month from now, you will have gained a lot of strength and can increase the amount of reps you do per set. Just stay consistent and you'll eventually get to where you want to be. Consistency and dedication always win out. So stick with it.

SUMMARY

What you've just read is a simple and very effective system for getting bigger, stronger, and also more ripped in the fastest, most efficient amount of time possible.

If you stick to using this system at home using bodyweight exercises during TV commercials and in mini-workouts, this is also the most convenient way to workout.

It's cheap. You don't have to pay for a monthly gym membership to do this. However, you could definitely do this system at the gym. The key to making this work for you is to make working out as effortless as possible, unless otherwise stated. The more effortless it is; the better.

You don't want to struggle doing the workouts. In fact, struggling hurts your results and progress. Simpler and easier are generally better for results.

Remember the following:

1. Never go to muscular failure… always avoid fatigue (unless otherwise stated).

2. Do a lot of sets with low reps (even though you can do more reps per set).

3.   If you're doing multiple sets in a workout, keep your rest times short.

4.   Make sure the exercise is challenging you and intense enough, but not hard or overly intense.

5.   Since your muscles and Central Nervous System are always fresh with this type of working out, more is better (as long as you follow the guidelines). The more volume (sets and reps) you can get in each week, the quicker your progress will be in getting bigger, stronger, and more toned up.

Within one month of doing the Effortless Exercise System five to seven days a week for at least 20 minutes a day, you'll see a transformation of your body in the mirror.

I encourage you to do even more than the bare minimum to get even faster and better results. One hour a day using this system would be great.

Think about how people will look at your differently in the future. An improved, stronger, bigger, and more ripped looking body changes the perceptions people have of you if you were out of shape to begin with. You'll get more respect from people of both sexes. You'll be more attractive to women. You'll have more confidence in yourself.

In short, you can open up a whole new world for yourself by following this system.

Change yourself, change your reality. A new and improved *you* will soon appear before yourself in the mirror. It's yours for the taking. You just have to take action and make it happen.

Good luck. Take care. Make yourself a better you and make this world a better place.

Sincerely,

Rich Bryda

P.S. Starting on the next page I include bonus reports that help to expand on the concepts in the Effortless Exercise for Men book. My goal with these reports is to provide added details to give you a clearer picture of the system and what you have to do.

Of course, there will be *some* overlapping and redundant information. This repetition is for your benefit to help ingrain what is necessary.

My bonus book, *Brute Force Push-Ups* follows!

BONUS BOOK:

**BRUTE FORCE PUSH-UPS
HOW TO DO 100 PUSH-UPS EVERY DAY
AND BUILD A POWERFUL CHEST
IN 1 MONTH**

BY RICH BRYDA

Introduction

I'm going to show you a simple program on how to easily build up to doing 100 push-ups each day and in the process develop a powerful chest.

I was always strong. I built up to doing a 435 pound bench presses in college. But the problem was that it did nothing for building up my chest. My chest wasn't impressive in my opinion. By doing all that benching, incline benching, and so on, all I did was build up my shoulders and triceps. That happens to a lot of guys.

You may move a lot of weight on the bench, but it doesn't translate into making your chest look nicer and bigger.

Once I put my ego aside and didn't worry about lifting as much weight as possible (or even lifting weights), then I was able to build my chest up really fast. And I did it surprisingly with only push-ups and burpees. This report focuses on push-ups, but you can use the same principles with burpees as well. So the good news is that you don't even need to touch any weights or go to the gym to build a bigger, better looking chest.

The goal for this program and the results focus on two things:

1. Get a bigger, more impressive looking chest.

2. Easily be able to do 100 pushups every day.

That's it.

I have a challenge for you. It's simple. Just do what I'm about to show you for 30 days. Take a picture of your chest before you start day and then take another picture of your chest on day 31. On day 31 your chest should look a lot better and you'll be able to easily do 100 push-ups a day by then.

I don't know you and I don't know where you're starting at as far as doing push-ups, but I'm going to teach you an "effortless" way to build up your push-ups strength while developing a big, alpha male, intimidating chest. If you're a beginner or way out of shape and can't even do 5 push-ups, then yes, it probably will take you longer than a month to be able to effortlessly do 100 push-ups a day.

Please be fair and realistic. If you follow this program, you'll rapidly progress with push-ups without struggling. Just put in the time.

The good news, if you're a beginner, is that most guys do push-ups wrong. So even advanced guys will have to go back and do push-ups the proper way… which means they won't be able to do as many push-ups as they think.

TESTING

You need to test your one-rep max with push-ups for a set. Do as many as you can until you can't do any more. This will give you a baseline to work off of during your push-ups workouts. You need to know what your max is in order to know how many push-ups you'll be doing for each set (since you can't go to failure).

But Wait!

I assume you're doing push-ups wrongly and that's probably the main reason why you don't think you'll get results or haven't gotten results from push-ups. A lot of guys can get a lot out of push-ups even by doing them wrongly… look at guys in the military. They do a ton of push-ups the wrong way, but still end up failing to build up their chests.

Anyway, here are the finer points of push-ups that you *must* keep in mind while doing this program. Following these tips will get you the most out of this program and your push-ups.

1. Your hands need to be out wide… wider than shoulder width apart.

This puts the emphasis on the chest and *not* your triceps. If you want push-ups to make your triceps bigger, do pushups with the thumbs of your hands no more than six inches apart.

2. Tighten your abs.

This is so the chest is the only part of your torso that touches the ground or comes close to touching the ground.

3. As you are pushing yourself upward, try to pull your hands together.

This is probably the most important thing about push-ups that everyone gets wrong. By doing this, you create incredible chest stimulation.

Now, to be clear, your hands won't actually move together when trying to bring them together. That's impossible without lifting them up. The goal is to get a great squeeze and contraction in your chest. So mentally and physically, you need to concentrate on trying to move the hands together. But they won't actually move.

However, you can use furniture sliders and your hands would move together. This is very advanced though. All you'd need to do is put your hands on the furniture sliders while doing the push-ups and pull them together.

Here's a link to the furniture sliders I use (again, you don't need these, it's optional) (this book's links are *not* affiliate links): http://www.amazon.com/Miracle-Movers-Piece-Furniture-Slider/dp/B003GU2MSY/ref=sr_1_13?ie=UTF8&qid=13256 17716&sr=8-13

4. Push yourself as high as possible.

Most people simply don't lock out and go as high as possible to do a complete, full-range repetition. This is very important.

Don't do half-reps by not locking out your arms and going as high as possible.

If you're able to do all four of the things above and still can do at least 20 push-ups, then what you will need to do is elevate your feet onto a bed, chair, or whatever in order to make it harder.

In conclusion, figure out how many push-ups you can do to the point of not being able to do anymore push-ups.

The Goal

The goal is to do 100 or more push-ups a day, every day. I'll soon show you how to do this easily and quickly so it's not a pain to fit into a busy schedule. What you want to do to make this as simple as possible while still getting great results is to *do half the amount of push-ups per set* as your maximum amount of push-ups that you just tested.

So if you can do 20 push-ups, then do sets of 10 and follow the "effortless" principles outlined above. So you'd end up doing 10 sets of 10 push-ups for the day. If you can only do 10 push-ups, then do sets of 5. So you'd end up doing 20 sets of 5 push-ups. If you can do 6 push-ups until failing, then do sets of 3 pushups. So, 33 to 34 total sets.

The goal is to do these sets of push-ups without struggling. If you're going to do all the push-ups in one workout, then rest 30 to 60 seconds between sets. If you're doing 10 sets of 10 push-ups; that will take you no more than 12 minutes.

One of my personal favorite ways to do push-ups is to do two sets during TV commercial breaks. So once a commercial comes on, I immediately do a set. Then I rest 30 to 60 seconds and do one more set. After that, I wait until the next commercial break to do two more sets. By doing it like that, I'm easily able to do all 100+ push-ups during one TV show that is 30 to 60 minutes long. You don't even sweat doing it like that.

After one week of doing 100+ push-ups each day, you will probably be able to add 1 to 2 reps to each set you do. So if you're doing 10 sets of 10 push-ups on the first week, then on the second week you'd end up doing 9 sets of 11 to 12 push-ups. Then on the third week you'd do 8 sets of 12-13 push-ups. The fourth week you'll be able to do 7 sets of 14 to 15 push-ups. This will save you time and provide extra stimulation to your chest.

If you continue to do 100 or more push-ups a day beyond the first month, then always try to add 1 to 2 reps per set each week while also decreasing the amount of sets by one. Just remember, it doesn't really matter how many sets or reps of push-ups you do or when you do them. The main thing that matters is that you do *at least* 100 push-ups *every day* for at least a month.

If you do 100 or more push-ups every day for one month (that is more than 3,000 push-ups), then your chest will get bigger. This works best for beginners and guys who think they're intermediate weightlifters, but advanced guys would also benefit by following this protocol. This is simply the best way to build up your chest. Yes, it's simple. But it works.

For advanced guys, no, this won't increase your bench press. If you want to increase your bench press, then you can use the neural imprinting method to grease the groove of the bench press and increase it that way. But for push-ups, we're greasing the groove of push-ups.

After you do a month of these 100 push-ups a day, you can either stop doing the push-ups and go back to what you normally do for the chest or continue doing 100 push-ups a day. It's your choice. After a month however, then you can start taking one day off a week. This means you'll only need to do the 100 push-ups for six days a week, not seven days.

You may think push-ups are easy and a joke, but if you did 100 of them a day for one month, your chest will be bigger. *I guarantee you!* I hope you try and prove me wrong because a month from now your chest will be bigger.

You can thank me then.

One last warning: *Don't* do any other exercises for your chest during this one month. The volume of push-ups is all you need. So if you want a bigger chest, all you need to do is *just do it*; do 100 push-ups a day for one month. That's it.

BONUS BOOK:
BRUTE FORCE PULL-UPS
HOW TO DO 20 PULL-UPS & BUILD A WIDE & POWERFUL BACK IN 1 MONTH USING THE "EFFORTLESS" PULL-UPS SYSTEM

BY RICH BRYDA

I'm assuming you already know what pull-ups are. If not, it's when you hold a bar and pull your body up so your chin goes above the bar. The palms of your hands are facing away from you. Chin-ups are when the palms of your hands are facing you. For building your back, you want to focus on *pull-ups*, not chin-ups.

Anyway, if you want a bigger, wider, more powerful looking back while being able to do twenty or more pull-ups for a set, then you've come to the right place.

If you get a big back, then you're big. It's that simple. Big chest, big arms, and big legs can get covered up and minimized in clothes, but a big back is hard to cover up. This is true in just about any clothing, even in a sweater.

Start Where You Are

I don't know you and I don't know where you're starting at as far as doing pull-ups, but I'm going to teach you an "effortless" way to build up your pull-up strength while developing a big, alpha male, intimidating back. If you're a beginner or way out of shape and can't even do 5 pull-ups, then yes, it probably will take you longer than one month to do 20 or more pull-ups for a set.

> **Note:** Please be fair and realistic. If you follow this program, you'll rapidly progress with pull-ups without struggling. Just put in the time. Also note that there will be overlapping and redundant information between my Effortless Exercise for Men book and this report. This is for your benefit to drill the information into your mind.

TESTING

You need to test your one-rep max with pull-ups for a set. Do as many as you can until you can't do anymore. This gives you a baseline to work off of during your pull-ups workouts. You need to know what your max is in order to know how many pull-ups you'll be doing for each set (since you can't go to failure).

Now, there are two programs to choose from.

The first program is for guys who are able to do pull-ups six days a week at the gym or home. If you can get a pull-up tower for your home, do it. It'll be one of the best investments in yourself you ever made. Guaranteed!

The goal for pull-ups at home is to do 50 or more daily. This equates to 300 a week.

> **Note:** Relax! I don't expect everyone to be able to do that the very first week. That's the goal you're shooting for. If you can already do 10 or more pull-ups for a set, then you should have no problem doing 50 or more pull-ups a day or 300 each week.

If you can do 5 to 9 pull-ups for a set, it may take you one or more weeks to do 50 or more pull-ups a day and 300 a week. If you can't do five pull-ups for a set, then it may take you two or more weeks. But don't worry. Follow the system and you'll increase your pull-up strength really fast.

The second program is for guys who can only workout at the gym. For this program, you'll need to do pull-ups four days a week and also 300 a week. At the gym, you'll need to do 75 pull-ups for each of four workouts. That's your goal.

The goal for each set of pull-ups is to do 25 to 50% of your one-rep max set of pull-ups. That's the "sweet spot" for neural imprinting with bodyweight exercises. In fact, the more pull-ups you can do, the lower the percentage you should use. So if you can do 12 pull-ups for a set, then for each set of pull-ups, you'll do 3 to 6 pull-ups.

To give you an idea, I was able to build up to doing 28 pull-ups for a max set without ever doing more than 6 to 7 pull-ups per set. In fact, I usually did just 5 reps per set. Are you beginning to see what I mean by it being "effortless"?

This will be easy for you. You're not going anywhere near the amount of pull-ups you can truly do for a set.

By doing this, you're not going anywhere near muscular failure, which taxes your Nervous System too much. This allows you to shorten up your rest times so you can do more sets and get in more total reps in a shorter amount of time.

You'll remain fresh the whole time you're doing pull-ups.

Effortless Exercise System for Men

PULL-UPS AT HOME

You can do this one of two ways.

First, you can do the pull-ups during TV commercials. Each commercial is usually 2 to 3 minutes long. Within that time, you'll be able to do 3 to 4 sets of pull-ups. Your rest times should be short, anywhere from 30 to 45 seconds. Nothing longer.

If you feel you need a longer rest time, than you're not following the rules. You'll need to do fewer reps for each set. Remember, each set you do has to be between 25 to 50% of your one-set maximum for pull-ups.

Let's use an example of you being able to do 10 pull-ups. Assume you're watching some TV with commercial breaks. There are about 8 commercial breaks of 2 to 3 minutes for every hour of TV programming. With you being able to do 10 pull-ups, you'll want to do sets of 3 to 5 pull-ups.

It's best to start out at the lower percentage and do three-rep sets of pull-ups. Truly, the amount of pull-ups you can do for sets is to a degree, irrelevant. It is total amount of pull-ups you do in a day that matters. Focus on the goal of doing at least 50 pull-ups a day.

When the first commercial comes on you leap into action. You crank out a set of three pull-ups. You then rest 30 to 45 seconds and do a second set of three pull-ups. Then you rest another 30 to 45 seconds and do a third set of three pull-ups.

You're done. For now. Go back to watching your show. When the next commercial comes on, you repeat that.

You keep repeating that sequence of doing your three reps of pull-ups for three sets during each commercial break until you've done at least 50 pull-ups. So it will take you less than an hour of watching TV to do that.

Do you see how easy that was? You didn't interrupt your day at all. You didn't interrupt your TV watching time either. You used the wasted time during TV commercials to fit in your workout.

Simple. You didn't sweat. You didn't struggle. All the pull-ups were easy.

Now just stick with it and follow this plan for six days a week. If you truly want to be a badass, you don't have to stop with just doing 50 pull-ups in a day. Boost it up to doing 100 pull-ups a day.

That's easy too.

The only thing you need to be careful of with doing 100 pull-ups a day is elbow or shoulder aches and pains. Always pay attention to your body and the clues it gives you. If your elbows or shoulders are getting achy, go back down to 50 pull-ups a day. And if they're still achy, take a day or two off every once in a while.

Even with the best system laid out, problems can pop up. Work around them. The second way to do pull-ups at home is to do then whenever. There's no rhyme or reason.

Say you can do 10 pull-ups maximum for a set. If, as an example, you're going to randomly do pull-up sets throughout your day at home, then instead of doing three reps per set, I suggest you do five reps per set. That is 50 percent of your one-set max.

The reason you can go closer to failure is because you're not doing a set of pull-ups immediately after the first set. So, randomly do sets of 5 pull-ups whenever you get a chance. You can again do these sets during TV commercials, just one per commercial if you want. I've found doing them during TV commercials is the easiest way to consistently do them. Just set up a routine. Make it a habit. This way you won't miss days or forget about doing the pull-ups until the last minute, late in the day.

Paper Helps

I've found that having a piece of paper with the amount of sets of pull-ups I'm going to do for the day listed helps a lot. Let's say you're doing 10 sets of 5 pull-ups for the day. Write on the top of the piece of paper "5 Pull-Ups Per Set." Then write the numbers 1 to 10 and circle each number. Once you do a set, cross out that number.

If you're going to randomly do sets of pull-ups without doing them during TV commercials, you may want to find a routine.

Maybe do one set right when you wake up. Cross that one out.

Then you do a set after you eat breakfast. Cross that one out.

Then you do a set before you leave for work. Cross that one out.

Three sets are now already finished. You get home from work and do another quick set. Cross that one out.

Keep this up. You could also do something such as this: every time you walk by your pull-up tower, you do a set. Make it a habit like that. Or after every time you come out of the bathroom, you do a set of pull-ups. Do it however you want. I personally prefer doing them during TV commercials for simplicity and to make it an easy routine to follow out of habit.

PULL-UPS AT THE GYM

Okay, you're going to have to do these four days a week at the gym. That is at least 75 pull-ups during each workout. There are two ways you can fit them in.

First, you can do your normal workout, but after each set of whatever you're doing, you do a set of pull-ups. So say you're doing bench presses. Do a set of benching then immediately walk over to the pull-up bar and do a set of pull-ups. Keep jumping back and forth between sets of whatever you're doing with sets of pull-ups until you've completed your 75 or more pull-ups for the day.

The second way is to do the pull-ups at the beginning of your workout. Do lots of low rep sets (25 to 50% of your one set pull-up max) with short rest times of 30 seconds. Say you can do 10 pull-ups for a max set. Then you'll do say three reps per set. For 75 total pull-ups, you'll need to do 25 sets.

Do a set of three, rest 30 seconds, do another set of three, rest 30 seconds, and so on. At this pace you'll do about six pull-ups per minute. So the total time to do all 75 pull-ups will be around 13 minutes or so. It doesn't take long. And it'll be really easy because you're never fatigued since you never go close to muscular failure.

That's all there is to it.

Effortless Exercise System for Men

RECAP

A review should be helpful.

Figure out your starting point. You'll need to first test yourself to find out the maximum amount of pull-ups you can do for one set. Once you know that, then you'll be able to figure out how many pull-ups you do for each set based off doing 25 to 50% of your best set of pull-ups.

If you're doing sets of pull-ups back to back, try to stick closer to the 25% for all your sets. If you're more random with doing the pull-ups and not doing sets of pull-ups back to back, then you can move closer to the 50% of your best set of pull-ups for all your sets.

If you're doing pull-ups six days a week, then do 50 or more each day. If you're doing pull-ups four days a week, then do 75 or more a day. You need to do a minimum of 300 pull-ups each week. It doesn't matter how many sets it takes you to do the 300 pull-ups. Just focus on getting in the 300 pull-ups each week even if it means doing 300 sets of one pull-up.

> **Note:** Trust me. You'll get a bigger back and a lot stronger from doing sets of a single pull-up as long as you do a lot of sets.

Just remember: Always follow these five rules and you'll be able to "effortlessly" get a bigger, more powerful V-taper back and should be able to build up to doing 20 pull-ups for a set in one to two months.

1. Never go to muscular failure during a set in order to keep your body fresh (for bodyweight exercises like pull-ups, try to do working sets of 25 to 50% of your maximum set)

2. Do a lot of sets of pull-ups

3. Do low reps

4. Short rest times (30 to 45 seconds)

5. High frequency (six days a week if possible)

If you follow these rules you can't help but to get a bigger back while building up the maximum amount of pull-ups you can do for a set. The great thing is, you won't find this to be difficult. It'll be easy. How do you know it'll be easy? Well, if it's not easy, then you're not following the rules. It's designed to be easy.

Good luck!

BONUS BOOK:

**HOW TO GET A SIX PACK FAST
GET RIPPED ABS WITHOUT DIETING IN
AS LITTLE AS 10 MINUTES A DAY AT HOME**

BY RICH BRYDA

I don't know where you're starting from, but if you use the tips I'm about to share with you, in a month, you'll either be shredded or getting close. Now, if you're 50 pounds overweight, obviously it will take longer, but in the first month you may feel better than you have for years and you'll certainly look better.

If you use this information consistently, I have no doubt you'll achieve your goals. You're probably extremely busy and have tons of responsibilities, right? That makes it hard for you to get to the gym to work out or spend extra time in the kitchen cooking up healthy stuff. These days it's hard to get ripped up.

Foods are loaded up with MSG, aspartame, preservatives, pesticides, hormones, antibiotics, and a whole range of other man-made chemicals that are destroying your health and making you fatter. This makes it seem virtually impossible to lose weight.

A Common Misconception

A common perception is that getting ripped abs is 80% diet and 20% exercise.

Nothing could be less accurate.

You *can* out-exercise a moderately bad diet if you know what you're doing. You *can* get ripped up while eating bad foods. Now of course it would help if you ate healthy, but I'm going to show you some powerful exercises that you're probably not doing that can put you on your way to *ripped city*.

What I'm about to show you is simple, but it isn't necessarily easy. You'll need to put in a lot of work and be consistent. But if you do that and give me 10 to 20 minutes a day of your time, six days a week, you'll develop a body that makes women desire you and other guys jealous.

There are 168 hours in a week. I don't care how busy you are, you can spare one to two hours of those 168 hours to exercise. That's around 1% of your time for the week. You can even do these exercises during TV commercial breaks. See, I'm making this ridiculously easy for you to do and make a habit of it.

The Routines

I'm going to outline five exercises here. You don't need to do all of them daily. In fact, you can stick with just doing one exercise each day if you wanted to. Some of the exercises get better and faster results than others, but they all serve a purpose.

I'm not going to give you a set routine to do. That's for you to decide. Each person is different. Do what suits you best. I will however make some suggestions. It's simple. Just do one or more of these exercises six days a week for 10 to 20 minutes. That's it.

Don't over-think this. *Just do it!*

Here we go…

The T-Bar Kettlebell Swing

If I were to pick one single exercise to get ripped up fast without even needing to leave your home, this would be it (Ok, maybe burpees is it, but this is a close second). This is the *only* exercise you'd need to do to drop a lot of weight *and* develop an ass of steel. You'll get better abs and a better ass, two of the top things women physically like in men. On top of that, it also helps improve sexual performance in bed.

Do I have your attention?

Below I'm showing you a picture of a kettlebell swing.

However, instead of a kettlebell, I want you to make a T-Bar Kettlebell because this allows you to adjust the weight. You won't have to buy multiple, expensive kettlebells.

A *T-Bar Kettlebell* costs about $15-20 in parts that you can get at Home Depot or Lowe's in the USA. If you're not in the USA, your local hardware store will have the parts you need. I'll explain more in a minute.

Here's the picture of kettlebell swings.

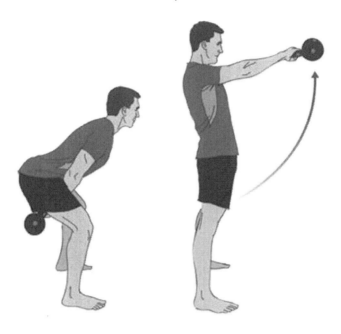

The finer points are hard to explain but simple to show you. Instead of writing about them, I'll link you to online videos.

Tim Ferris, author of The *4-Hour Body* has two videos. The first video shows you how to do the swings properly. The second video talks about the T-Bar Kettlebell as a cheap replacement for swings instead of kettlebells.

http://www.fourhourworkweek.com/blog/2011/01/08/kettle bell-swing/

The two keys for swings are to stick out your butt and then thrust your hips forward. You don't want to use your arms and shoulders to muscle up the weight. Use your butt and hips to power the weight up through the swings.

In the picture above, the form is slightly off because he's raising the weight too high and extending out his arms too much which will cause your arms and shoulders to muscle the weight up.

Keep watching the videos until you understand these key points so you'll know how to do swings correctly. Now, the second video doesn't give enough details on how to buy or create your own T-Bar. So I'm going to expand on that.

When you go to Home Deport or wherever to buy the parts, write this down on your list:

- A 3/4-inch x 10-12 inches long galvanized steel pipe nipple (if you are normal height or taller, go with 12 inch long pipe; if you're shorter, go with 10 inch long pipe). This will cost about $4.

- 3/4-inch by 4-5 inch long galvanized steel pipe nipple (you need to buy two, these are the handles you'll hold on to, so make sure you get two and not one). You can get a 4 inch pipe, a 4.5 inch pipe, or a 5 inch pipe. I recommend a 4.5 inch pipe if possible. That works for people with average or slightly big hands. If you have really big hands, get the 5 inch pipes. Two of these pipes will cost $3-4 total.

- A 3/4-inch galvanized steel T coupling (this is to connect all 3 of the pipes above to each other). This costs about $2.50.

- A 3/4-inch galvanized steel Floor Flange. This will be the bottom part of the T-Bar, which will hold the weights on so they don't fly off while you're doing the swings. This will cost about $6.

- A 1-2 inch spring clamp. This will cost $2-3.

The total cost for everything is less than $20.

To put this together, all you do once you have all those parts is to screw the three pipes into the T coupling until they're tight. You only need your hands. Then screw the Floor Flange to the bottom of the 10 to 12 inch steel pipe. Make sure the Floor Flange is extremely tight. You don't want the weights flying off.

All of this takes about two minutes to do.

You can then remove the handle part by unscrewing it with your hands. Then you can slide weight plates on. That's the genius behind the T-Bar as a replacement to kettlebells. Your one T-Bar can be any weight you want it to be. You can add or remove weights as you wish.

You'll need to buy *standard* weight plates separately. I don't know how strong you are, but if you're average strength or pretty strong, you might want to start out with 30-50 pounds of weights. Get a bunch of 10 and 5 pound plates.

You can also get 25-pound standard (not Olympic-sized) weight plates from Walmart for about $20 each. I prefer you get 10 pound weights because they're smaller and easier to swing between your legs. Practice your form on the swings with just 25-30 pounds to begin with (or less if you feel that is too much weight).

Once you have your T-Bar Kettlebell and you have your weights, what then? Here's what I suggest you do in order to lose a lot of weight and get ripped up:

Pick a weight, anywhere between 25 and 50 pounds and simply do 200 T-Bar swings a day for six days a week.

That's it!

Now, you can do this however you want. It doesn't matter how many swings you do per set. Just do a total of 200 swings however possible. The first few times you do this you'll probably be extremely sore. After the first day of doing 200 swings, you'll probably want to rest a day or two.

Then in two to three days, do another 200 swings. If you're really sore again, then take another one or two days off. After that, you should be able to do them every day, six days a week.

Here's how I recommend you do the 200 swings for a workout. Do them all in 15 to 20 minutes. Try to do sets of 15 swings. Make an effort to build up to that if you need to.

Keep doing this workout every day and trying to beat your best time. Try to get it so you do 200 swings in about 12 minutes. Once you can do that with whatever weight you were using for 200 swings in 12 minutes or less, increase the weight by 10 pounds. This will make the exercise harder and it'll take you a little longer to do. But again, keep trying to beat your best time and once you can do this new weight for 200 swings in 10 to 12 minutes, increase the weight again.

Continue that progression. Also, if you're main goal is simply to lose weight and get ripped up and you're not an athlete training, I recommend that you don't go over 100 pounds with the T-Bar swings. You can if you want, but I recommend that you don't.

A second way you can do your T-Bar swings workout is to do the swings during TV commercial breaks. Watch a typical one-hour or 30-minute TV show. Then during the commercials, do your swings. The typical one-hour TV show has 7 to 8 commercial breaks that last about three minutes long. So that's plenty of time to fit in 200 swings while allowing you to watch TV and without messing up you schedule.

Note: Make sure dogs, cats, wives, and children are out of the way! A hit with a kettlebell isn't quickly recovered from.

The bottom line is that if you're able to do 200 T-Bar swings in 10-15 minutes a day, six days a week, using a decent amount of weight (50 or more pounds), you honestly don't even need the rest of the tips in this report in order to lose weight and get ripped up.

The swings alone are all that you need. In fact, I hope you start out by focusing only on doing the swings and nothing else. This makes things as simple and uncluttered as possible. You don't have to mentally think about anything else.

Now, your next exercise…

5 Minute Star Runs/Walks

This is right up there with the T-Bar Kettlebell swings as far as losing a lot of weight fast and getting ripped up. If you have stairs in your home, then it's even possible to do this without leaving your house. This exercise is extremely simple and straightforward.

What you do is run as fast as possible up 1 to 3 flights of stairs. Then you walk back down them. Keep repeating that sequence over and over for 5 minutes. The key to this is to not stop. Keep moving. You'll get your rests on the walks down the stairs. Stair Runs/Walks require an active rest, not a passive rest.

This is another exercise that you can do alone without any other exercises for fat loss. You'll be able to see results in the mirror *within* two weeks just doing this exercise 5 to 6 times a week for five minutes each time.

Now, will you be able to do this the first time you try? Probably not, unless you're in really good condition already. If that's the case, and you can't do the full five minutes of running up the stairs and walking down them, then you'll want to slip in some walks up the stairs.

As an example: Run up the stairs, then walk back down the stairs, then the next time up the stairs you walk up them to give you an extra bit of rest. Then you walk down the stairs. Then you run up the stairs. Maintain that sequence. Essentially, that sequence is every other time up the stairs you will walk instead of run. In fact, the first time you try this exercise, you may want to just walk up and down the stairs for five minutes non-stop to see how it goes.

Then mix in a few runs up the stairs the next workout. Keep doing that until you build up to only running up the stairs instead of mixing in walks up the stairs. Another thing to remember is that the Stair Runs/Walks are great for preserving your muscle mass while helping you lose fat. (The same can be said for the T-Bar kettlebell swings too.)

This top-of-the-line fat loss exercise produces better results than just about anything else. If you don't have stairs in your home, go find a building nearby that does have stairs. The only drawback for this exercise is the fact that a lot of people can't do it in their home.

> **Note:** Finding stairs makes this routine less convenient than the T-Bar kettlebell swings. That's the only reason I rank this below T-Bar kettlebell swings. But you'll see awesome results from both.

Stair Runs/Walks may be too much of a hassle for some people. And when that happens, they aren't consistent and skip out on doing the exercise. Doing that ends up compromising results. Regardless, if you can do the stair Runs/Walks, then add it in and do it.

If you're already doing the T-Bar kettlebell swings six days a week, then doing the Stair Runs/Walks 5 to 6 days a week may be too much for your body to handle. Don't think you have to do both six days a week. If you can manage that, definitely do it, but if not, it's okay.

Burpees

Want to know the secret to how convicts locked up in prison are able to get jacked up without using weights while eating crappy food?

Burpees are their secret. Yes, I'm back to talking about burpees. I may annoy you with the redundant information, but I'm fine with that because I want to emphasize this exercise.

Burpees make you bigger, stronger, more ripped, and also build athleticism into your body. Getting bigger and stronger doesn't help as much as people think when fighting. If you don't know how to move your body fluidly during the fight you'll likely to lose no matter how strong you are. So burpees offer an added benefit and an additional reason why convicts put a lot of focus on doing burpees.

Here's how to do burpees:

1. Begin in a squat position with your hands on the floor in front of you.

2. Kick your feet back while you go down into a pushup.

3. As you're pushing up with the pushup, return your feet into the previous squat position.

4. Jump up as high as you can from the squat position.

5. Keep repeating, doing them as fast as possible.

Not only will you get a bigger chest from doing these, but you'll get ripped up fast and get in great condition while gaining muscle mass all over your body.

There's a reason why prisoners do burpees all the time. Burpees work and they do so much for you beyond simply getting bigger and stronger. I don't know what your conditioning level is or what your athletic ability is, but definitely try to incorporate these into your workouts.

The routine's goal is simple: Work up to doing 100 burpees in less than 7 minutes. Now, you probably won't be able to do that to begin with. So what you'll want to do is sets of 5 to 10 burpees. Rest 30 to 60 seconds between each set and do a total of 100 burpees. (If you can't do that because of your conditioning, then rest a little longer.)

> **Note:** If you can't do that because you can't do five burpees, then just practice doing burpees until you can do sets of five burpees.

The progression you'll want to use is to do 100 burpees in less time. That's your goal for each new workout if the goal is to get as ripped up as fast as possible. You can do this by adding 1 to 2 burpees to each set. This will allow you to do fewer sets in order to do 100 burpees. Once you're able to do 10 burpees per set, then the progression you should use is simply to lower your rest times between sets.

It helps if you are wearing a watch that has a stopwatch feature so you can accurately time your rests. I use a $15 Walmart watch and it's great.

To illustrate the proper way to do burpees, I did a quick Google search so you can see a video of how to do them. Here's it is:

http://www.youtube.com/watch?v=c_Dq_NCzj8M

If you can do 100 burpees a day, five to six days a week, that's great. That's the goal that you should shoot for in order to get shredded. But again, if you're mixing and matching exercises from this report, that may be hard to do.

Doing 200 T-Bar kettlebell swings, 5 minutes of stair runs/walks, and 100 burpees a day is simply too much for most people. You should divide everything up throughout the week as you get stronger.

>   **Note:** If you want to try doing all three, then your best bet is to do them separately in three short workouts.

By doing that, you'll get an idea on what your body can do and handle.

Tabata Jumping Jacks

I know, you probably think jumping jacks are a joke. I did too. But that's because there are a few key things you weren't doing when you did jumping jacks. If you use the proper workout protocol and you seriously put effort into them, jumping jacks will beat you down.

First off, I don't put tabata jumping jacks in the same category as the above three exercises. But this is a good option to help you get ripped at home.

Tabata is a form of interval training. Tabata requires just four minutes of your time. But it's an extremely intense four minutes, even with simple exercises. It becomes 20 seconds of exercise followed by 10 seconds of rest. You will keep repeating that for a total of four minutes.

> **Note:** You need to be *precise* with those times for this to be effective. Too many people turn 10 second rests into 20 to 30 second rests.

This exercise format is really intense and you can use it for a whole bunch of other exercises too. I recommend that you do this twice a week to change things up from the other exercises listed here. This means it will take you just 8 minutes of your time for the whole week.

The entire concept is named after Dr. Tabata who discovered that this type of interval training produces much better fat loss results than aerobic training. It's not even a close comparison. In fact, four minutes doing the Tabata interval is equal to doing 45 minutes of normal cardio training!

You may want to read that again because it's profound and revolutionary.

The four minutes of doing Tabata intervals may feel like the longest four minutes of your life too.

Here's how you do them.

You can do almost any exercise for Tabata intervals, but in this case, I recommend power jumping jacks. You should do them as fast as possible for 20 seconds non-stop. Then you rest 10 seconds. You will repeat them doing as many power jumping jacks as possible for another 20 seconds and resting 10 seconds.

Keep repeating that until you eventually stop when four minutes are over. You'll do 8 total sets. Try to be as accurate as possible with your timing. If you have a stopwatch feature on your watch or phone, use that. Or if you have a clock with a moving hand, do this exercising while watching the clock. I personally use a Gymboss timer.

Just remember the key: Do the jumping jacks as fast as possible. Don't do them slowly! This isn't meant to be a casual exercise. You're going to take an easy exercise like jumping jacks and make it hard and effective for fat loss.

Just in case you want to see how to do jumping jacks, here is a quick video I found through a Google search:

http://www.youtube.com/watch?v=dmYwZH_BNd0

Note that the video's star did not do the jumping jacks explosively or as fast as possible. You however will. That is the key to making jumping jacks effective. You will do them explosively and as fast as possible. I can't stress that enough. By doing that and using the Tabata Protocol, you'll get quite the mini-workout for fat loss.

One more exercise remains.

Medicine Ball Slams

Medicine ball slams are a great cardio workout that will help you develop some crazy abs. As with most great things, it's simple and straightforward. You pick up a non-bounce medicine ball, lift it over your head, and slam it down into the ground as hard as possible.

The key to making this effective for getting your abs stronger and more ripped is to do them fast and with as much power as possible. If you don't put that effort into them, then your results will suffer.

Here's a video I found on YouTube that shows you how to properly do medicine ball slams:

http://www.youtube.com/watch?v=ARbWy62ZMWw

I have no clue who that guy is and I'm not promoting his stuff, but as far as medicine ball slams go, he teaches them correctly. You'll need to use a non-bounce medicine ball because if you use one that bounces, it will ricochet back into your face. That is anything but pleasant.

Here's the link to where I bought my non-bounce medicine ball:

http://www.xtrainingequipment.com/Slammer-Ball_p_17.html?gclid=CNz_yZHK8KoCFdMS2god5VzINA

Medicine balls definitely aren't cheap. But if you can make it happen, it's definitely worth buying. Since you probably have never done medicine ball slams, I suggest you start out by getting either the 20 pound or 25 pound medicine ball.

For most guys, that's about right. It's not too heavy and it's not too light.

As you advance and the 20 or 25 pound medicine ball becomes too light for you, you may want to move up to a 35 or 40 pound medicine ball. But honestly, that's not necessary. You don't need to buy a bunch of medicine balls. This is exactly why I showed you how to make your own T-Bar Kettlebells, so you don't have to buy a bunch of different kettlebells that are different weights.

What you will do is this: Do 100 slams in less than 15 minutes.

In subsequent workouts, try to do the same amount of slams in less time. That's the progression to use.

100 or more slams in 15 minutes or less is simply a suggestion. Don't be afraid to get creative and do your own thing.

A workout I really like doing is 15 T-Bar Kettlebell swings immediately followed by 10 medicine ball slams without rest. After I'm done with the medicine ball slams, I then rest about a minute and repeat that sequence.

I keep doing that for a total of 15 to 20 minutes.

A Complete but Quick Recap

So to recap: You don't need to do all five of these exercises each day or even each week to get ripped up. You can just focus on one of them and do it daily. Or you can mix and match a couple of them. If you can break things up into two very short workouts a day, that works even better.

Perhaps try something like 10 minutes of T-Bar Kettlebell swings for the first workout and then a second workout four or more hours later of about five minutes of Stair Runs/Walks and five minutes of medicine ball slams.

Get creative. I don't want you to feel limited to doing things just one way. Use this guide as just that, a guide.

I can guarantee you one thing. If you seriously put effort into the exercises listed in this report, you can't help but to get more ripped up. And the results come fast. You simply need to put in the effort. I'm not asking much of you. It only takes 10 to 20 minutes a day. If you need to use TV commercial breaks, that's fine. Do that. Get the work in however possible.

You don't need to go on some special diet either. Eat like normal. The only change you need to make is to do these exercises.

Go make it happen.

You're so close to getting ripped.

Effortless Exercise System for Men

BONUS BOOK:

BRUTE FORCE BICEPS WORKOUTS HOW TO GET BIGGER ARMS (1+ INCHES) IN 1 MONTH AND ONLY 4 WORKOUTS

BY RICH BRYDA

If you follow this simple workout routine once a week for four weeks, in a month you should have arms that are at least one-inch bigger than they are today.

I've developed and tweaked this routine to perfection from testing on myself and others. It's common to gain 1/2 inch on your arms after the very first workout (although you'll have to wait one to two days to see that size gain). Some guys have gained over two inches on their arms in a month using this workout.

What I want you to do is measure your arms so you know your starting point. Then don't measure your arms again until you've completed this workout once a week for four weeks.

Keep It Short and Effective!

Now, this report is not a comprehensive book on getting your arms bigger. You won't learn a ton of arm exercises or workout routines. This is exclusively focused on your arms to gets results fast and in only one day a week. Nothing else is needed.

Although everything here is simple, it's not easy.

One thing you're going to realize is you probably can't do this on a day you're working (unless you work from home and control your own schedule). You'll most likely need to do this on an off day. I encourage you to do this on a Saturday or Sunday. If you're a huge football fan, this is perfect during the fall. In fact, as you'll see, the workout revolves around football for me.

The only equipment you'll need will be a set of dumbbells. That's it.

Now, if you say "But I don't have dumbbells," the logical and obvious answer to that would be: go get a set of dumbbells. The main workout can and should be done at home, but just in case you can't or won't get some dumbbells to use at home, I'll give you an alternative routine you can do at the gym.

If you have a choice between doing the home workout or the gym workout, choose the home workout. Your chance at success is higher due to how easy it is on your schedule.

Triceps Too

Don't let the name of this report fool you. Part of the routine is an exercise that targets the triceps. Why is that? It's because the triceps make up 2/3rds of your upper arm size. If you want bigger arms, you can't neglect them and just focus on the biceps. It's a complete workout for your arms.

Now let's get started.

Effortless Exercise System for Men

ARM WORKOUTS AT HOME

Soon you'll have bigger arms to add to your bigger chest. You don't need to leave the house to do it.

Rule #1

Pick a day that you don't have to work and have a lot of free time.

As you'll see, the workout at home isn't a traditional workout. In fact, you need to spread it out throughout the whole day. You'll be doing this on and off for six to ten hours.

Rule #2

Use TV commercials.

The workout consists of four sets done within two minutes, multiple times a day. Since most commercial breaks are two to three minutes long, they are perfect to use for these mini-workouts. By using commercials, it makes it easier on you to do the workout without thinking too much.

There are usually around eight commercial breaks per hour. So they pace the workout for you.

The two great things about using commercials to work out are that you can sit there and watch TV. You don't have to sacrifice TV time for workout time. You can do both. Also, working out during TV commercials doesn't interfere with your relaxation or schedule. Commercials are usually wasted time for people. You can put that time to good use.

During the fall, at least for Americans, there is football all day on Saturday and Sunday. If you love watching football, then it's perfect to squeeze in this arm workout while you're watching football. This obviously works only during football season.

Regardless, just pick a day where you have a lot of free time.

Rule #3

You can only do this arm workout once a week.

Don't even think about doing it more than once a week. It's a simple workout, but it's not easy. In fact, it's quite brutal. It's going to test your manhood. Now, if you can't or don't want to do it once a week, but instead maybe do it every once in a while that's fine. Do what you can and what you're comfortable with. Once a week isn't always possible.

And you definitely don't need to do it once a week, every week, for a year or longer. Once a week for four weeks is more than enough. After you do that, then wait another two months before trying it again. Use this as a "shocker" workout to shock your arms into growing.

Rule #4

Expect extreme soreness in your arms for at least one to two days after doing the workout. Basically, you're going to hate me the first couple of days after you do the workout. Your arms will be like hanging slabs of meat. Keep that in mind when you plan out your workout days. You won't be able to work out for at least two days after doing the arms workout and simply moving your arms might be quite painful.

The reason for the soreness is because you'll be creating severe muscle trauma to the triceps, biceps, and brachialis muscles in your arms. You need to do this in order to get your muscles to "super-compensate" and grow.

No pain, no gain. Remember how I said there are many different ways to get bigger and stronger. Well, this is one way that is *not* effortless.

Now, one thing I want you to be prepared for is that it's possible you will *temporarily* lose size in your arms. *Relax!* Don't worry. It's only temporary and part of the super-compensation process. A day later your arms will *explode!*

The reason why your arms will probably shrink for the first 24 hours after the workout is because they'll be completely depleted of glycogen.

This leads to the next rule…

Rule #5

Eat a lot the next day or two.

You'll need to eat and drink a lot. A lot of protein, a lot of fats, and a lot of carbohydrates the day after you do the workout. Your body, specifically your arms, will need this nutrition to rebuild and repair for the growth that's about to happen.

Eat like normal during the workout (remember, it's over the course of 6 to 10 hours), but after the workout, eat a lot of food. Make sure to get a lot of carbohydrates to help replenish your glycogen levels.

THE EXERCISES

There are three exercises you will do in this program. They are...

- Normal dumbbell biceps curls

- Hammer curls

- Diamond pushups

These exercises alone aren't anything special. They get the job done. They're the tools you need. But it's the workout structure, timing, and volume that are what makes this program so special.

Dumbbell Biceps Curls

I assume you know what normal dumbbell biceps curls are, but just in case you don't know, here's a video of them:

http://www.bodybuilding.com/exercises/detail/view/name/dumbbell-bicep-curl

Obviously, this targets your biceps. Be sure to curl up both dumbbells at the same time.

Hammer Curls

The reason hammer curls are in this program is because they target the brachialis. This part of your arm is often neglected. And it's a big reason why so few guys have big arms.

If you don't know where the brachialis is on the arm, it runs underneath the biceps and helps to push up the height of your biceps. It's basically the bump between your biceps and triceps on the outside part of your upper arm near your elbow.

Your arms need to be developed to notice it. You can do a google search for "brachialis" if you want a picture.

To target the brachialis, we'll be using hammer curls. Here's a video of hammer curls:

http://www.bodybuilding.com/exercises/detail/view/name/hammer-curls

For hammer curls, be sure to do one arm at a time, unlike normal biceps curls.

Diamond Push-Ups

They're called diamond push-ups because your hands are close to each other to the point where your index fingers and thumbs are nearly touching each other.

The open space between is in the shape of a diamond, or a triangle.

Normal push-ups are great for the chest, but to target your triceps, you need to bring your hands in closer together for push-ups.

Here's a video of diamond push-ups:

http://www.bodybuilding.com/exercises/detail/view/name/push-ups-close-triceps-position

Effortless Exercise System for Men

THE WORKOUT

Now that you know the exercises that you'll use and the background information, here's the workout:

1. You will do 100 total sets for the day.

2. You'll do these sets during TV commercials.

3. You'll do four sets during each TV commercial break and a total of 25 different mini-workouts during TV commercial breaks in 6 to 10 hours.

4. 6 to 8 diamond push-ups

5. 6 to 8 dumbbell biceps curls (using a 10-rep max weight)

6. 6 to 8 diamond push-ups

7. 6 to 8 alternating hammer curls (using same weight/dumbbells as biceps curls)

Do the mini-workout in that order. *Don't change* the order of the exercises.

It's only four sets.

When a TV commercial comes on, do those four sets in that order. Try not to rest between the sets. But the main goal is to get all four sets done within the timeframe of the TV commercials, which are normally 2 to 3 minutes. If you can't do 6 to 8 diamond push-ups, then do what you can. You probably shouldn't even do this workout if you can't do at least 10 diamond push-ups.

For biceps curls, you'll be doing 6 to 8 reps for each set, but use dumbbells that you can curl for 10 reps. You don't need to go to failure. The volume will take care of muscle growth.

For hammer curls, you'll use the same weight that you used for biceps curls.

Recap

Let me lay it all out for you.

You'll have 25 mini-workouts of four sets. There are about 7 to 8 TV commercial breaks per hour. *Don't* do this workout every commercial break. Ideally, you'll do each four set mini-workout once every 2 to 3 commercial breaks. At the start you'll probably want to do it every other commercial break. Then after a few hours you'll probably want to extend your rest between each mini-workout so you do them once every 3 commercial breaks. That'll average out to about 3 workouts per hour. Finish up all 25 mini-workouts of 4 sets in 6-10 hours.

To keep track of how many sets you're doing, I suggest you get a piece of paper and write the numbers 1 to 25 on them. Each of those numbers will represent one four-set mini-workout.

After each four-set mini-workout you do during a TV commercial break, cross off a number.

That's it. Get ready for your arms to burst.

ARM WORKOUTS AT THE GYM

Unfortunately, not everyone can work out from home. That's fine. I'll show you a version of this workout you can do at the gym.

It's the same 3 exercises:

1. Diamond push-ups

2. Dumbbell curls

3. Alternating dumbbell hammer curls.

The two differences in the gym workout will be that you do fewer sets and do everything in one big workout as follows:

Do one set of 6-8 diamond push-ups. Without rest, immediately do one set of 6 to 8 dumbbell curls using a weight you normally can do for 10 reps. Again, without rest, do a set of 6 to 8 diamond push-ups. Then after that, without resting, do a set of 6 to 8 hammer curls.

You'll end up doing four sets in a row without rest.

After you do those four sets, rest two minutes.

Then keep repeating that four set sequence followed by two minutes of rest for a total of 15 times. This means you'll end up doing a total of 60 sets. It should take you about 45 minutes to complete everything.

Towards the end of the workout you may not be able to do the full 6 to 8 reps. If that's the case for the diamond push-ups, then just do as many as you can. If you can't do 6 to 8 reps for the curls or hammer curls, then you can reduce the weight slightly in order to do the full 6 to 8 reps.

Do this gym workout for your arms just once a week.

It doesn't matter which arms workout you do, the gym one or the one at home. I prefer the home workout; others prefer doing it at the gym. Either way, your arms are going to get a lot bigger. Also, you can switch back and forth between them and one week do the workout at home and the next week do the gym routine. If you can't do the workout to begin with, then build up to it. Just do fewer sets.

In Conclusion

So there you have it.

You only need to do three exercises to gain up to a half inch on your arms after just one workout and one or more inches after four workouts. And you only have to do one workout a week. What could be simpler? If you have a set of dumbbells at home, then this is perfect to do at home. If not, use the gym routine. Good luck!

Rich Bryda

P.S. Read below on how you can get a free surprise gift...

Effortless Exercise System for Men

BONUS GIFTS!

As a special thank you for buying this book, you can get the following 10 reports free at my website here: http://WeightLossEbookStore.com/bonus

1. *How to Lose Weight Spinning in a Circle like Kids*

2. *The 20-Second Bathroom Trick for a Super-Charged Metabolism and a Flood of Energy*

3. *One Tablespoon of this $6 Supplement Detoxes 900 Yards of Toxins from Your Body*

4. *Do-It-Yourself Face-Lift: How to Look 5 Years Younger in 2 Weeks – Got 5 Minutes a Day?*

5. *The 50-Cent Miracle Weight Loss Food You're Not Eating*

6. *#1 Cheap Supplement that Reverses Gray Hair & Infuses Health into Your Body*

7. *How to Get Rid of Allergies in 90 Seconds with Water*

8. *The Ultimate 3-Second Fountain of Youth "Neural" Fat Loss Exercise*

9. *The 15-Second "T-Tap" for Overcoming Hypothyroidism & Sluggish Energy*

10. *How to Make Healthy Ice Cream in 2 Minutes and Other Sweet Surprises!*

ADDITIONAL GIFT

If you decide to take just a few minutes to write a review for this *Effortless Exercise System for Men* book package on Amazon, I want you to immediately email me the review confirmation email Amazon sends you to socialmediapublishing@yahoo.com so I know you left a review. Once I see that, I'll email you a special surprise gift. Trust me, you'll like it.

> **Note:** I am not asking you to write a 5-star review in return for the gift (although I'd love it if you felt the book along with all the bonuses were worthy of 5 stars). What I am asking you is to please write a thoughtful, productive, and fair review.

Sincerely,

Rich Bryda

socialmediapublishing@yahoo.com

Made in the USA
San Bernardino, CA
22 February 2014